THE MAN WHO MOVED THE NATION

THE MAN WHO MOVED THE NATION

WHO
MOVED

A DAUGHTER'S STORY

LISA JENNIFER COLLINS

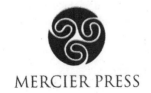

MERCIER PRESS

MERCIER PRESS

Cork

www.mercierpress.ie

© Lisa Jennifer Collins, 2018

ISBN: 978 1 78117 570 5

10 9 8 7 6 5 4 3 2 1

A CIP record for this title is available from the British Library

Printed and bound in the EU.

CONTENTS

JUNE 2013

1 I Really Don't Have Time For This   11

2 Say What Now?   23

3 What The Hell Is Happening?   35

JULY–AUGUST 2013

4 Making A Plan   47

5 So It Begins   58

SEPTEMBER–OCTOBER 2013

6 Life According To Chemo   69

7 Reflection   77

NOVEMBER 2013

8 State Your Business   89

DECEMBER 2013

9 I Don't Know If I'm Cut Out For This   105

10 Are You Home Yet?   114

11 The First Ad   122

12 Christmas   133

13 Here We Go   141

JANUARY 2014

14 We've Won   149

15 Famous   155

FEBRUARY 2014

16 Respite   169

17 The Hospice   182

MARCH 2014

18 We Need To Talk About Gerry   193

19 Goodbye Dad   202

Epilogue   207

Family Notes   213

Acknowledgements   220

For my father
and
my husband.

Thank you for everything.

JUNE 2013

1

I REALLY DON'T HAVE TIME FOR THIS

'Lisa, it's your dad. I'm in St Michael's in Dún Laoghaire. I need you to do me a favour.'

I'm standing in my bedroom with a towel around me, the phone to my ear. I turn the music down so I can hear him better. *What's he doing in there?* He never mentioned he had a hospital appointment coming up.

'They're saying they need to keep me in, so I need you to bring me in some clothes. Are you around?'

Some clothes? Keep him in? What for?

I stand very still. 'Yeah no problem,' I reply. 'But what's going on? Why are they keeping you in?'

'I'm not really sure, honey. They're saying there is something wrong with my lung.'

Inside, my heart beats out of sync and my stomach tenses and releases at the same time. On the outside I stay calm. The word *lung* has shocked me and automatically I veer away from it.

'Oh God. Are you okay? I'm sure it's just your ribs again, Dad. They probably haven't healed properly yet. Honestly, you'd think in this day and age they'd be able to do more with broken ribs. It's absolutely ridiculous.'

I hear him hesitate. 'Yeah, maybe. Honestly, though, this is a total nightmare, Lisa. I have a meeting with an important client in an hour. I really don't have time for this.'

I'm not surprised to hear him say this. He's self-employed and business is business. I understand that; I'm self-employed, too. There's no time for being sick when you work for yourself.

'Dad, don't be worrying about that, that can wait. The important thing is that you are properly checked over.'

I can feel his agitation at the situation through the phone. 'Yeah, yeah, I know, I know. Your brother dropped me in very early this morning for a quick check over as I had a bit of a "thing" on my run; I really didn't expect them to keep me in, and now I'm in a hospital bed.'

A 'thing', he says. I'll get more on that later.

'Just bring me in my trackies, my white M&S T-shirt, my toothbrush, and whatever else you think. You know.'

I try to take in what he's saying, but this is all a bit odd. It's also strange that I'm getting this call and not Mum. She's usually the person who would be the first point of contact for things like this, but they aren't exactly on speaking terms right now. I reassure myself: *It's okay. I can do this.*

'Grand, Dad, no worries, I'll be in with them in a few hours, I just have a couple of clients to see first.'

'Thanks, honey.'

I hang up and put the phone down on my dresser. I stare at it, trying not to overthink things, but my mind keeps throwing me back five years to when I got the news he had throat cancer.

Not again. Please. Not again.

I feel sick.

***

After grabbing the few bits for him from his place, I drive to the hospital. By now, I'm annoyed. Typical Dad. Thinking about work instead of his health – though it is something of which I too am guilty. I remember an incident a few years ago when Dad and I were working on a project together. One day he and I were in the car on the way to a client meeting when we stopped at a roundabout. Without warning a large Range Rover drove into the back of us. The guy just wasn't looking. Dad ended up in hospital and I should really have gone as well, but both of us were in shock and so, at the time, it didn't strike either of us that it was a bad idea for me to go ahead to the meeting. In hindsight, it was obviously not a good idea. I arrived at the meeting dishevelled and still clearly shaken after the accident. I'd say the people I met must have thought I was insane given that I was babbling a hundred miles an hour at them about sponsorship, all the while looking as pale as a ghost. But shock can do funny things to a person.

As I take the exit for Dún Laoghaire and St Michael's Hospital, adrenaline is making me giddy. I need to release some of this energy. I pick up my phone, put in my earpiece and call my friend Becki.

'Hey, what's the craic? How did Saturday night go?' I ask, just wanting to talk about something trivial.

'Great laugh, Lis. After you left, we went upstairs to the nightclub, danced the legs off ourselves and crawled into bed around three.'

I smile. Good woman, Becki. This is why I called her. She loves to burn up a dance floor and is a great wing woman for giving it loads on a night out. Normally, we'd barely have a drink. Don't need it.

As she fills me in more on what happened last Saturday night, I start laughing, even though nothing particularly funny has been said. Suddenly I become aware that I'm driving too fast and should probably slow down. Better to 'Arrive Alive', as the ad says.

'So, what are you up to?' she asks.

'Not much, hun; just heading into Dún Laoghaire.'

'Cool, what's going on there?'

I'm reluctant to tell her, afraid to make something out of what's probably nothing. Still, I do. 'I'm just dropping some clothes in to my dad. He's in St Michael's. He went in this morning for a check-up of some kind and they kept him in. To be honest, Becki, I'm not really sure why he's there. He did mention his lung.'

'Oh God, Lis!'

'I'm sure it'll be grand.'

My tone is confident, yet I know I am fiercely pushing back a contradictory pitch.

'I hope he'll be okay,' Becki says.

A wave of panic threatens to wash over me. Lung and wrong – they don't belong in the same sentence. I get a feeling of pins and needles in my arms. I rub them to get rid of the sensation. There is no evidence to say anything is seriously wrong, I frantically reassure myself. But this doesn't help when my gut is telling me that I don't need evidence, that we've been here before.

'I hope so too, Becki. I hope so too.'

***

I pull in to the hospital, not knowing where to park. There are roadworks everywhere and the car park is a building site. Somehow I manage to throw the car into a tight spot. Dad would have applauded my precision. It's not an official car space, of course, and I hear a few roars from the builders, but I don't care. I just want to get in and see my dad.

Once inside the hospital, I go straight to the receptionist and ask for my dad's whereabouts.

'He's in the far wing,' she tells me.

As I walk along the hospital corridor, I continue in my efforts to keep myself calm. *Right, there is no emergency here and there is no urgency here.* Still it takes all my strength not to burst into a full-blown run. I smell the hospital smells, so sterile and overpowering. Memories from past visits start rolling through my mind. My grandad, my mum's dad, was here a lot in his later years. I used to visit him quite a bit, so I'm familiar with the building.

I manoeuvre around elderly people in the corridor and

negotiate my way past a cleaning trolley. I just need to get to my dad. I am sweating by the time I get to the nurses station.

'Excuse me, do you know where Gerry Collins is?' I ask as I take off my hoodie. 'He came in this morning.'

'Let me check,' the nurse says, flipping through a clipboard. 'Ah yeah, Mr Collins is down in room 16A, just there on the right.'

'Okay, cheers.' I'm happy knowing he's only metres away.

I walk more slowly now, trying to calm my breathing, which has been thrown off by my anxiety, so I won't look panicked when he sees me – even though my heart feels like it is trying to escape through my chest. When I reach the door of 16A, I take a final slow, deep breath and put a smile on my face. Then I push the door open and walk in.

There he is. Sitting upright in the bed. He's got a white T-shirt on, which he must have been wearing under his suit this morning. He's reading a book. Nothing new there. Some Irish history book, no doubt. Dad eats books for breakfast, lunch and dinner. He looks up at me, smiles and puts the book down, taking off his reading glasses.

'Ah, you're an absolute pet; thanks a million,' he says.

I look around. It's a private room, he has it all to himself. It's nice and bright and he has a fabulous view of Dún Laoghaire bay. I sit down at the end of his bed and pass him his sports bag with the things he asked for in it. He doesn't even go through the bag. He's just happy to have whatever I've brought in and to see me.

'You did well for yourself getting this room, Dad. Who did you have to pay for this view?'

He laughs. 'You don't want to know what I had to do to get this room.'

That's how we work. We laugh through difficult times in our house. We will get to why he is in here in a moment, but we both know this chit-chat is necessary; it allows both of us time to adjust.

'Well at least you have a book. That's good, thank God you're not in here with nothing to do.'

'Yeah, couldn't be in here all day without anything to read. I got this book a couple of hours after I was admitted. I really didn't expect to be kept here, so I had absolutely nothing with me. I asked the nurses could I run over to Eason's across the road when it opened, but they said I couldn't leave the hospital now that I'd been admitted.'

My spidey senses tingle. I feel certain by his tone, and the slight smirk on his face, that he has definitely been up to no good. I can see from here that, without a doubt, the book is brand new. So he's either charmed the nurse herself to go get it for him, paid some passer-by or swindled it somehow. I am half smiling myself now, with one eyebrow raised.

'Oh? So how'd you get the book?'

'I went over myself! I just waited for the nurse to leave, jumped up, threw my clothes on, grabbed €20 from my wallet and legged it over.'

'Daaaad!'

He's smiling at me with both his eyebrows raised as if to say, 'You gotta do what you gotta do.' Dad never was one for the rules. That's something I really love about him. He's his own man.

'So, I found this book, jumped straight to the top of the massive queue, waved the book at the lady and put €20 on the counter before darting back to the hospital.'

He laughs heartily, cracking up at his own antics.

'It was gas; they could see the hospital band on my wrist as I waved the book at her.'

He has me cracking up now too.

'I nearly got caught though.'

So there's more!

'As I was going back towards the room,' he continues, 'I could see the nurse ahead, so I went into the toilet and left the book up on the windowsill. I just walked out of the toilet then and she found me. "Gerry," she says to me, "I've been looking for you." "I was just in the toilet," I said.' He's laughing so hard now that tears are watering his eyes. 'She made me get back into bed but I grabbed the book after she left and here I am!' He slaps the book in his lap.

We laugh again until we don't. I have to ask.

'Right, so what's the story here, Dad? What happened?'

'Well, I got up yesterday to go for a run. I didn't feel great and my ribs were at me again but I thought it'd do me some good. So off I went but I only got as far as the second round-about before I collapsed. I found it very difficult to breathe; it was quite frightening, actually. I thought I'd better get the once-over and so I came in here this morning.'

The infamous rib situation. Dad trains in a boxing club in Camden Street three times a week and has done for the last four years. He's not actually supposed to be getting into the ring, as it's more about the exercise and breaking a sweat than actually training to fight. 'It's good for the head,' he constantly says. 'Healthy body, healthy mind, lads,' he'd say, even if he was talking to me and my sister. However, back in January he got into the ring and took a pretty hard blow to his left ribs. He ended up in Loughlinstown and there they discovered that two of his ribs had been broken.

It's now June, so the ribs should be healed, but from what I can see they haven't healed at all. He's been in a lot of pain since, with no sign of any major improvement. He's constantly holding his side.

'So what's the story? Is it your ribs then? Have they checked them out?'

'Yes, honey, they have. They took X-rays this morning. My ribs have totally healed.'

'Okay, well that's good. Phew.'

Finally. At least we know they're okay now. That's good news. I'll tell Mum, she'll be happy to know that. I can let my brother, Stephen, and sister, Ciara, know, too.

I'm the eldest of three. Next is Stephen and last but far from least is Ciara. As siblings go, we don't live in each other's pockets by any means, but we're very close on a deep family level.

But even as I think this, I'm struggling to hang on to my relief because I have a sneaking suspicion that it will be short-lived, as I've yet to hear about his lung. I'm not even sure what could be wrong. Like, what could it be? He's already had cancer, so it can't be that.

Dad's looking at me with a soft smile on his face. I'm feeling more frantic than I'd like to let on. My eyes dart around the room more than I'd like them to. He says, 'So, yes, my ribs are healed and that's good but when they had a look at the X-ray they could see that my left lung is full of fluid.'

What? Fluid? That's mad. Okay, how did that happen? I'm wracking my brain for diseases that cause fluid in the lung. *Pleurisy?*

'That's why I've been struggling to breathe and that's why I collapsed when I went for my run.'

That makes sense.

'So, when I thought it was my ribs that were hurting me all this time, it wasn't; it was my lung. It just happened to be on the same side as the broken ribs, which was deceiving.'

I listen intently. Shit. I am probably staring at him pretty sternly right now, I realise. It's my 'okay, we have a problem but we will fix this' face; it tends to look stern. I'm not sure if I've even blinked since he mentioned fluid in his lung.

His voice raises a notch. 'So listen, the nurses have been great and they are coming back shortly to drain my lung and do some more tests.'

I don't like the sound of this. *Drain his lung?* He's still smiling and I know he's trying to be comforting. *How are they going to do this and more tests for what?*

Seconds later, a middle-aged male nurse comes in holding a clear plastic cylinder about a metre in length and quarter of a metre in width. There's a long tube coming out of it at the bottom. He also has a tray with him which looks like it's holding different-sized needles. *Oh God. What are these for?* This is all moving so fast.

'Okay, Gerry, let's get the lung drained and you feeling better.'

The nurse looks at me and explains that he's about to insert a needle through Dad's back to start the draining process.

I am *not* good with needles and blood. The last time I was in a hospital was in April during my stay in Guatemala for Stephen's wedding. Ciara got sick and we had to take her to hospital. I stayed with her in the treatment room while they took blood, only to wake up on the floor after passing out. The mortification; I was meant to be holding *her* hand. My blood pressure dropped and I ended up in another bed beside her hooked up to a drip. It was a disaster.

Looking at me looking at the needles, Dad says, 'Okay, honey, you really don't need to stay for this.'

He knows.

He puts his legs over the side of the bed now and gets into a seated position facing the window. The nurse pulls over the wheelie tray and positions it in front of him. He asks Dad to lean forward and try to breathe normally. So he's now sitting on the side of the bed, looking out on beautiful Dún Laoghaire harbour and is about to have a giant needle inserted through his back, threaded between his ribs and directly into the lung. This all seems so sudden and savage for someone who was just admitted this morning. I am holding back tears now.

The nurse is getting all his utensils lined up on his tray.

'Honestly, go, love, it's grand,' Dad says. 'This won't take long and I'll be fine then. I'll give you a call after. Honestly, it's better they don't have to drag you out of here by your legs after making a holy show of both of us,' he laughs.

I look at him and nod. I have no words; I can't speak.

I pick up my bag, give him a hug and make for the door. I turn back to look at him and he's facing out the window again, his back to me.

I want to stay!

As the nurse starts to insert the needle, I think: *this cannot be happening!* Then I whisper goodbye and slip out the door, trying and failing to absorb what is currently happening to my dad and the fact that I can't stop it.

2

SAY WHAT NOW?

I'm waiting for my first client of the day. I have the wax on, melting, my bed set up. The place is warm. It is summer, so the sun hits the window around 10 a.m. and heats the room naturally, filling it with light. I put the music on. I just love it here; this is my happy place. I work hard in my studio and the hours are unsociable, but it doesn't feel like work to me. When I tell people what I do for a living their response can be, 'I don't know how you do your job, waxing body parts all day', but my reply is simple: 'I don't know how you can do your job, sitting at a desk and looking at a computer all day!' To be fair, waxing probably is a bit of a calling, but if that's the case, then I have been called!

I opened Wax It Studio about a year ago, in July 2012. It was a big decision to leave the security of employment and a guaranteed monthly pay cheque, but it was one of the best decisions I ever made. I had started out as an event organiser navigating the corporate world, moving later into the hotel industry as a corporate sales manager. The experience and mentoring I received from some of the fantastic people alongside whom I had worked over the years proved crucial when I was setting up my own business. Sometimes I laugh when I see the files I have saved on my laptop. In particular, in my sales and marketing folder. My current 2013 strategy is already in place and I'm working on 2014 with an overview of 2012 to hand to remind me what tactics worked well before and should be repeated. If my folder represented my studio it might be easy to assume I'm trying to take over the world, but basically it's just me in a room and I love it.

The best thing about my work is my clients. They make my day every day. I meet great people here, and I hear so many of their stories and feel privileged that they share them with me. In many ways I go on their life journeys with them, especially my female clients. I might hear about a new man they've met, an engagement, their big day, a pregnancy, fertility issues, deaths and pretty much every other life event. That's what it's about for me: connecting with people on a real level.

The next best thing about my studio is that I can be myself. Before, when I put that suit on every morning and headed for Dublin at 7 a.m., a blanket would come down and smother me. The real Lisa Collins faded and another Lisa Collins, 'suited and booted' for corporate life, was pushed to the fore. It was exhausting. So I founded Wax It Studio and created a new world, a world in which I looked like me, sounded like me and acted like me. It allows me to breathe more freely.

There were other changes, too. I moved into a three-bed duplex in Greystones, which was a mere ten minutes from my studio. This marked the beginning of my friendship with Kat, with whom I share the house. Our place isn't the most orderly, but it's a fun and peaceful place to be. We recently hung photos in an effort to make it feel more homely. I've never seen anyone hammer so many nails as I saw Kat do that day. And all in less than five minutes! Kat the enthusiast. The homelier the better, she says! And that duplex is home now, a girlie place littered with scented candles, comfy throws and long chats.

The buzzer goes and I am shaken back to my present.

Donna, my first client, comes through the door. Donna. Guaranteed laughs for thirty minutes. Generally we bounce off each other. We both think the other person is hilarious. We are each other's biggest fan. Today, though, I'm not feeling funny. I hope she's up for talking more than me.

Dad is constantly on my mind. He is still in hospital, awaiting the results from the fluid they removed from his lung two days ago. They're testing it for everything. The suspense simmers constantly beneath every act and conversation. It seems wrong to even be working right now. I just keep thinking of him, lying in the bed, waiting and not knowing. That said, there has been a glimmer of light amidst all this awfulness that has filled me with a great sense of relief: Mum visited Dad yesterday to see how he was.

I am so happy about this. I don't know how much she is going to be around, but if Dad needs help it appears she is considering being a point of contact for him medically. She looked pretty concerned when I drove out to her after leaving Dad in St Michael's. I know she was thinking the same thing as me – something wrong with his lung equals something bad. I know she was remembering 2008, when Dad was diagnosed with stage-four throat cancer.

It's been four years since any of us had to give serious thought to cancer and Dad. Four years from those awful hospital memories. We learned our lesson that time. We all realised the fragility of life, and now we embrace it and each other. We cling together. We don't need to be reminded. We appreciate each other, love each other. *We are good! Please leave us be. Please.*

It can't be easy for Mum. Her and Dad have been separated for the last two years. It was a shock when they broke up. Although they are quite different in their make-up, I certainly didn't see it coming. After twenty-eight years, you kind of assume it's forever. When they separated, the family home was sold and they both moved into separate apartments. Handily, both are not far from where I live. Dad in particular is only about a two-minute walk away.

Since then, we have had separate Christmases; two Christmases that have been laced with sadness and with the dawning realisation that things were going to be like this from now on, that every Christmas myself and my siblings would have to deal with the same awkward questions. Do we have breakfast with Mum and dinner with Dad this year? Or do we have breakfast with Dad and dinner with Mum? Either way someone is left on their own.

I hate it.

Things are still not great between Mum and Dad. They are angry with each other and usually only talk if absolutely necessary. That said, when Stephen got married in Guatemala a few months ago, we all flew over for the wedding and during that time Mum and Dad very much rose to the occasion and were united for Stephen and Karina's big day. I had found it weirdly inspiring, watching them. However, since then they haven't spoken – that is, until yesterday. So I don't know how it's going to pan out, but I do know what I'm hoping for.

Six clients come and go. Donna started the day well for me and so the day flies by. I text Dad to see how he is.

'Just finishing this chapter,' he replies, 'then off to sleep.'

One more sleep for all of us before the results come in.

***

I wake up in surprisingly good spirits. In a weird way I am looking forward to hearing the test results today. At least we don't have to wait weeks – that would kill us. The waiting is the worst. I feel optimistic that this will not be as bad as we all fear.

Later, I message Dad, telling him I am heading in to him and asking if he needs anything. He replies and says he's grand, that the doctor is due at 2 p.m. *Perfect*, I think. I will be with him when the doctor arrives.

When I arrive into St Michael's I head straight up to Dad's room. As I draw near I can hear Dad laughing. His laugh makes me smile. I walk in. There he is, sitting up in the bed, chatting to his friend John and looking just like Dad should – bright and happy. To me, this is a good sign. What they did for his lung must have helped. He is laughing hard now, telling John about his Eason's escapade. John is clearly finding this as hilarious as Dad does. The two of them are cracking each other up. The laughter is infectious and I join in.

John is a great friend of my dad. They became friends later in life, through Toastmasters, and bonded further over music. I particularly like John because he has been very supportive over the last couple of years and has really shown that he has Dad's best interests at heart. John is a few years younger than Dad, though Dad slags him for having greyer hair than him. Do you have a friend with whom, no matter what is going on in life, you will always find the humour? Well, that's Dad and John. Of course, they drive each other mad too, and can spark off each other, especially when it comes to their beloved band – The Upbeats – and who is singing what song!

The Upbeats were born after Dad got 'kicked out' of a previous band. It's quite the story, really. He started playing the guitar properly about three years ago. He had banged around on it over the years, but could only ever play three songs: 'The House of the Rising Sun', 'Country Roads' and 'Little Old Wine Drinker Me'. They were his three songs for as far back as I can remember. Every Christmas those songs would get an outing. Every party those songs would get their moment. However, after he recovered from throat cancer, he decided to take the guitar by the strings and learn how to play it properly. So, just as he always does, he put 110 per cent effort and practice into it, and after a few months of playing every day (and wrecking my mother's head) he started to get pretty good.

Along the way he heard about some music sessions that were happening in Dún Laoghaire, where people would get together in a pub and play their various instruments, conducting sing-songs that they may have practised during the week. He started doing this every weekend and it really helped his confidence; as he'd say to me, it 'filled up the tank with the good stuff'.

It was at one of these sessions he met a guy who played in a band and at some point Dad joined them. Some of these guys were seriously talented musicians. Dad loved the idea that playing with them meant there'd be more demanded of his own playing. Typical of Dad, though, once he'd fully committed he soon wanted the band to grow, to get 'big', and so he wanted them to practise endlessly. He wanted to take the band to what he thought was the next level. He endeavoured to ensure that everyone knew every single word to every song they played, so that no one should be referencing or glancing at song sheets. God forbid! In short, Dad tried to take over. Well, his good intentions backfired and they 'kicked him out'.

I couldn't help but laugh when he told me.

'Can you believe it?' he'd said, disgusted. 'They actually kicked me out!'

I found his disbelief endearing because he should have known by then how he can be his own undoing sometimes. 'I don't blame them, Dad, I'd have kicked you out too,' I said, laughing down the phone.

'Well, it doesn't matter. I'm going to start my own band!'

And so off he went and did exactly that.

John, Dad and a few others set up the new band. Initially Dad wanted to call the band Gerry and The Upbeats. Unsurprisingly the other members didn't share his enthusiasm, so after some discussion a consensus was reached to call the band The Upbeats.

The Upbeats comprised a group of guys, some of whom had never played outside their bedroom, had never performed in front of any size of audience on any stage and certainly had never played alongside other musicians in a band. Dad organised weekly practice sessions and he played with a couple of them individually outside of 'practice' hours to help build their confidence. And after a while they ended up playing in front of people. Dad liked to support people, whoever needed it, and would play louder to cover for someone if he saw that they were struggling. He would also single someone out and praise them in front of a crowd to help build their confidence, and would try to ensure that everyone got a chance to play their song.

That's what Dad can make happen. He has a gift when it comes to people. He has the ability to reach right through your chest, into your soul, pull out all your good qualities and hold them up for you and the world to see. After thirty minutes of talking to Dad, you could walk away feeling like you are good enough to take over the world.

***

As I sit at the end of Dad's hospital bed, I listen again to the rest of the Eason's story, delivered through bursts of laughter. I do love Dad's hearty laugh.

The doctor comes into the room. *Finally*, I think, *we can figure out what the hell is going on here*. I wonder what it is. I hope he won't be out of action for too long. God forbid he shouldn't be able to go boxing or play the guitar. He'd go mad!

We stop the laughing and the chatter. I mutter a 'hi' as the doctor walks up to the side of the bed, just ahead of where I'm sitting. Out comes the clipboard and she looks at it for a minute. I thought she was going to start going through it with us but instead she hugs it to her chest and looks directly at Dad.

'Gerry, we have your test results back.'

There's something about the way she speaks that puts me on high alert. She's speaking really clearly and slowly, like we are foreign and can't properly understand her. 'We examined the X-rays we took after we drained your lung. Unfortunately they have revealed a large tumour at the base of your left lung, which is not good news.'

Did she just say tumour? Large tumour? No way, lady. Back it up there right now. Don't be throwing that word around so loosely. I feel myself getting angry – most people's go-to emotion when they or someone they love is threatened. It's also my initial go-to emotion if I'm sad. So here I am, hearing the word 'tumour' and I can feel the anger beginning to seep in.

'A tumour?' I interject. 'What kind of tumour, like? There are many different kinds of tumours! Is it benign or malignant?'

Dad's foot touches my back. It makes me turn to look at him. His face is calm as he nods at me.

'Okay, well what's the state of play here, Doc?' Dad asks. He's so good in these situations. He makes it so easy for her to do her job.

'Well, Gerry, there are cancerous cells in the fluid we drained. I am not the consultant here so I cannot give you absolute confirmation of anything further until we do more tests, but I think it important that you know this is not good news.'

Oh. My. God.

My ears are ringing. I can't quite hear what she's saying now. She's looking at the clipboard and saying something else. I can't look at John. I can't look at her. I need to look away from this woman. I drop my head and stare at the floor. My eyes are blurring. *Jesus. Did she say cancer cells?*

'Okay. Am I in serious trouble here?' I hear Dad ask.

'Unfortunately, yes, Gerry. We're pretty sure you have lung cancer but we don't know how bad it is. From the X-rays, we can see that the tumour is at the base of your left lung and it has actually breached the lining of your lung, so it's very difficult to know if it has spread at this time. What needs to be done now is to patch up the hole that the tumour has caused. This will then prevent your lung from filling up with fluid again. This procedure is called Talc Pleurodesis and it needs to be done soon. We are transferring you to St Vincent's tomorrow morning and they will be taking care of you in their Oncology Department.'

Ah here. What is happening? Lung cancer? Operation? Patching his lung up? Although that doesn't sound like the worst idea. Maybe that's a good thing.

'I understand that, Doc, and thank you, but I need you to give me further confirmation right now. Can you give me some idea of what I'm looking at here? How long do I have left?'

Why the hell is he asking *that* question? He is so matter-of-fact about this. How is this possible? It's like he's already had weeks to digest this information. I continue to stare at the floor in horror, devastated that this question has even been brought up. I feel like someone has thrown me forward in time to a point where my world is completely different. A few days ago my biggest worry was where I was going out Friday night with the girls. Now this.

'All I can really say here, Gerry, and I am so sorry to say it, is that what the tests showed is really not good news.'

There she goes again. Not good news. Not good news. Not good news. Yeah, we heard you the first time.

I really wasn't expecting this. There must be some mistake here. This is not happening. *Breathe, Lisa, breathe.* On the outside I am sitting silently; inside I am a raging storm. *Please let this not be happening.*

'I hear what you're saying. Thank you,' my dad responds.

She nods and puts her hand over my dad's hand for a moment, for which I am grateful. Then she leaves.

I finally look at Dad. His face is soft. It's like he knew. He doesn't look shocked or scared. He is half smiling, though it's a sorrowful smile. I turn to face John now and he is reeling. 'I wasn't expecting this,' he manages to say.

I shake my head as the situation starts to really sink in and tears begin to trickle down my face. John hands me a tissue. I am so upset. My poor dad. I'm horrified at the thought that there is a large tumour inside him. We need to get it out. I'm looking at his chest now and imagining it in his lung – that rotten, rotten tumour.

'Let's see what the tests come back with before we panic here, lads,' Dad says.

He's right. We don't know exactly what is going on here and, until we do, we should not panic. We also need to be brave for

Dad. If I am finding the news hard to digest, how must he be coping inside?

Please, please don't let anything be seriously wrong with my person. I won't survive without him. I won't. I cannot be here, in this world, without him.

They need to fix this. They need to fix him. And they will. Yes, I can tell from what the doctor said that it will be a challenge, but we are a strong family and we will hold him up. We did it before and we will do it again.

I am coming back to myself a bit now. The ringing in my ears has stopped and so have my tears. I am not generally a dramatic person but that had been hard news to hear.

'You're right, Dad. We don't even know what she said actually means.'

I don't think what I said actually made sense but it's all I can muster.

Let's keep this in perspective. What we do know is that this is worse than we thought; it is not good news; there is definitely something quite wrong with his lung. So now we just need to know what we can do to stop it, mend it and fix it!

It's late in the afternoon and Dad is tired, so we leave him to sleep. It is all making sense now – why he was so tired all the time recently. Come to think of it, he has lost a lot of weight and there I was thinking he was just stressed out. God, I didn't even question his sleeping in the chair sometimes, assuming that's what older men did. Even though he isn't that old. He hasn't been eating well either, saying that he just wasn't hungry.

It was all there in front of us. We just didn't see.

3

WHAT THE HELL IS HAPPENING?

As I drive to St Vincent's Hospital on Merrion Road, I speak on the phone with my friend Louise and fill her in on what's happening. Over the last few days Dad has disclosed the situation to his side of the family and close friends. He is the eldest of four; his sister Rosemary is next in line, then Declan and Paddy. His mum has not taken the news well at all. I don't have children myself but it's not hard to imagine how frightening this must be for her. To hear that your child might be seriously ill is something most parents hope never to have to endure, regardless of their age.

Dad was moved to St Vincent's a few days ago. They're doing more tests and prepping him for his operation, which is happening tomorrow. It's all very surreal at the moment. No one knows quite what to say because no one has any real answers. Bits and pieces of information are filtering through and being passed around from one day to the next, like a game of medical Chinese whispers. There has been nothing yet about the plan of attack on the tumour; patching up his lung is the immediate priority. The procedure he is undergoing – Talc Pleurodesis – will involve two incisions, one through his back and one through his side. They will both reach through to the lung. Sterile talc will then be adhered to the pleura, which is the lining of his lung. This will stop it from refilling with fluid going forward and will make it much easier for him to breathe. He's been very breathless, so that will be a huge relief for him.

As I park the car, I say goodbye to Louise and make my way inside the hospital. My heart lifts when I see Ciara sitting in the ground-floor coffee shop, looking at her phone and drinking something from a Styrofoam cup – hot chocolate, no doubt. Ciara is six years younger than me and we are very close. Most people say we are the image of each other, though she has long blonde hair and I have short brown hair – well, I actually have very short hair on one side and slightly longer, jaw-length, on the other side.

She puts her phone down and I give her a big hug. I'm so glad she's here, though she looks on edge. But that's not surprising. I take my wallet from my bag and go grab a drink. We've all been hanging out between this little coffee shop and Dad's room for the last few days, hot chocolate and croissants being the main menu choices. The coffee guy is so lovely. His friendly and warm manner makes it feel like he's empathising with us. I wonder why a smile from a stranger can help sometimes? I have no answer. It just does. I expect I will eventually forget his face but I won't forget that he made us feel like he cared.

I sit with Ciara and we chat. It's interesting, how we're each trying to be useful in our own way, but no one knows exactly what 'useful' is in this situation. Perhaps it's not our turn to be useful; it's the turn of the surgeons. Waiting seems to be our main occupation for now.

I spot Nana and Rosemary walking in. Nana has aged fantastically and looks at least fifteen years younger than she is. She's a glamorous-looking woman; make-up, nails and hair always immaculately done. I remember as a young girl wanting to try on all her jewellery when I'd visit. I still do! Rosemary is very like her, though I think she looks more like her dad, who died of a heart attack about twenty years ago. I was seven when he died but I remember him well. We called him 'Gang Gang'. Not far off Grandad! All I ever wanted to do was play with him and he was so patient with me. He would take me off to Marley Park and let me run myself ragged, though looking back I suspect this was more a favour to my parents. Still though, he would let me jump on him and bring me out to help him with the gardening, showing me how to pot plants and weed beds. He worked for the Department of Agriculture; his garden was always beautifully pruned. My favourite part of the garden was a huge blossom tree out the front that, when in bloom, would make you stop to demand your appreciation. When it shed its flowers it was like the sky was snowing pink flakes. I only knew him for seven years, yet at times I still miss the connection I had with him.

Nana and Rosemary don't see us as they walk straight past. We don't bother to attract their attention as we're having a conversation on the medical information we know to date about Dad's situation. Soon enough we finish up and follow them to Dad's room.

We arrive upstairs, not far behind them, and peer into the room. Dad's in a six-bed dorm and finds the lack of privacy hard. He's meant to be in a private room but there's no space for him at the moment. If a room becomes available he will be the first to be moved. The current room is pretty crowded, not only with his visitors, but his fellow patients' visitors too. There are very sick, elderly men on his ward, who seem to be in a state of dementia or drug-induced restless sleep.

Dad, though he is apprehensive about the surgery tomorrow and detests being bed-bound, is somehow managing to keep a smile on his face. He deals with things by consciously focusing on the positives, so we try to reflect that back to him and keep our conversation light.

Today is Tuesday. We won't see him until Thursday, as he'll be too groggy for visitors after the surgery tomorrow. I hope the procedure won't be too hard on his body. Thankfully he's strong for his age, with an above-average level of fitness due to his boxing and healthy diet. In fact, the doctors have said that if he wasn't so fit he'd be in much bigger trouble right now. It just goes to show, if you take care of your body it can really help you out in a time of need. 'You have to put the right petrol into your body, Lisa, so it can go the distance.' Dad loves his car metaphors.

This is all a very different mindset from the life he led up to ten years ago. Back then he worked in recruitment, headhunting and wheeling and dealing. It was all about the 'scene' back then – out schmoozing with clients, drinking, smoking and eating crap food whenever he could grab something en route to the next deal he was trying to close. It was back in the time when you could smoke inside, which every smoker did.

I remember how in my final year of school, in 2001, I would often go to his office in Dawson Street in Dublin and wait for a lift home. I was completely fascinated by the people working there. Extremely glamorous and smartly dressed, it looked as if each person was on a mission to seek and destroy. The energy in the place was electric. There was a big brass bell in the centre of the large, open-plan office, which was rung loudly any time a 'sale' was closed, followed swiftly by the name of the person who closed the deal and how much they closed it for being scribbled on the whiteboard used to display how people were progressing towards their monthly targets. Cheering and clapping would swiftly ensue when the bell rang, with a celebratory cigarette immediately lit. I thought they looked so cool. Sometimes when Dad wasn't there they'd give me a cigarette too and I'd sit in with them and pretend I was one of the gang. At that time, in my young, very impressionable eyes, this life looked so impressive to me. How naïve I was.

Then, ten years ago – for reasons only known to him – he decided to completely change his life. He just stopped smoking. He had finally had enough. He went from a forty-to-sixty cigarettes a day habit to zero, completely cold turkey. He decided soon afterwards that drink was also not a positive factor in his life and so he let that go too. He started to educate himself about food and took some cooking courses. This started his road to a healthier diet and working out. Within a year he had completely changed his whole lifestyle.

Surely the life he led over ten years ago has not caught up with him now? He already paid the price five years ago with the stage-four throat cancer. Life couldn't penalise him twice. Could it?

The end of visiting hours comes and we ready ourselves to leave. As I give him a hug goodbye, I want to hold him for longer, as if this could be the last hug I give him. But I don't want to go there, so I just give him a normal hug.

'Right, Dad, I hope you sleep well tonight, now. You're in the best of hands here, so rest easy and we'll see you on the other side.'

'Thanks, pet, I'll be grand here,' he says, waving a new book he has acquired in the air. He nods at me and I nod back.

Everyone else says their goodbyes and we head off. We're all nervous but we can't let those nerves rise to the surface. PMA – Positive Mental Attitude. That's the key.

On my way out I say goodbye to the nurses at the nurses station. I need to see their faces. It's like when you're on a bumpy plane and you're wondering if everything's okay and so you stare at the air hostesses, looking for the slightest sign of distress. If they look even a tiny bit worried you know there's a good chance you might be fucked. Poker-faced or smiling – you know you're grand.

'Bye now, he'll be fine,' one of them says.

That's enough for me.

We head home to let the waiting commence. I start visualising the operation as being a great success. The incisions are small, swift and precise. The lung will welcome the procedure, taking the talc dressing well and healing quickly afterwards. I continue to visualise all this again and again and again.

***

It's Thursday and I cannot wait to see him. Mum phoned, having just been with him. He's been moved to St Anne's Ward. They're saying he should fully recover in about six weeks. Though the surgery went well, she's warned me that he's a little weaker than she expected and probably looks a little worse than he is, so I'm to prepare myself for that.

Yesterday was a long day. I called Dad before he went into surgery. He was in good spirits, though anxious to just get it done. He went in on time at noon but the procedure took longer than expected. Every minute that it ran over felt like an eternity. When he finally came out they assured us everything went well. Their words were welcome, though they did little to remove my apprehension.

As I head to St Vincent's, I feel a mixture of relief and sadness. That's the second invasive procedure in just over a week. There is a sense that the surgery is a positive thing, of course, because it will help him. But I can't help feeling sad about the fact that he's had to be cut open for *any* reason. After all, no one likes to see their loved ones in pain. I actively try to put the surgery in perspective by thinking about what the doctors might have done back in the day if something like this happened. They wouldn't have had the advanced medical training to perform a procedure like this, so he probably would have died.

Today *is* a good day.

When I arrive at St Vincent's I walk in and see signs for St Anne's Ward on the first floor. In an effort to remain calm I walk slowly towards the ward. It's a recovery unit, so it's much quieter than the last ward Dad was in. I notice a young woman trying to navigate a Zimmer frame towards the loo. She looks weak, yet alert. I'd say she won't be on that frame for long.

I turn a corner and see my uncle Paddy outside a room at the end of the corridor. He has his head down as he walks from side to side with his arms crossed. He looks up and gives a small wave but there is a worried expression on his face. He starts walking towards me and I am suddenly having trouble moving my feet. They feel heavy. I stop walking altogether. When Paddy gets to me, I'm just standing there, my chin quivering like crazy.

'Don't worry,' Paddy reassures me. 'Come on, he's fine. He's absolutely fine. He just needs time to recover but he will be fine. He's just down there. I'll bring you down.'

He gives me a big hug and puts his arm around me and we slowly walk to Dad's room. I suddenly feel like a little girl and am very unsure how to handle myself. There's a sudden reluctance in me to see him. Why is that? I've been so excited to see him, but right now I feel major resistance to walking into that room.

I get down to the bottom of the ward and stall again outside his room. I look up at Paddy and burst into tears. I just do not want my dad to be in pain and I don't want to see him like this.

Shit. Panic stations. My poor, poor dad. I don't want him to see me like this, either.

Jesus, Lisa, get it together.

Sorry, it's just all happened so fast. It's a lot to digest, in fairness.

Great, now I'm talking to myself.

'You're okay, go on in,' Paddy says, looking sympathetic.

The door opens and I catch a glimpse of Ciara, Stephen and Mum, who are there already.

I take a big deep breath and walk in.

Oh my God.

What has happened to him? He looks terrible. He's sitting in a chair with his dressing gown on. It covers all of him except for his left arm and side, which are exposed. There's a clear tube coming out from his left side, just at his ribcage, connecting to a bucket with a lid on it that has been placed on the ground. It's being held in with white sterile tape and I can see blood and fluid going through into the bucket.

Oh God, the blood. I know Mum had warned me, but I had expected him to look better than this.

He looks up and smiles as best he can. He's holding onto his side. He is very pale. 'Hiya, honey. How are you?'

I walk over and sit down beside him. Tears stream down my face. I wish I was stronger for him right now but my heart is breaking. Paddy sits on the high stool beside me.

'How are *you*, Dad?' I manage to get out.

'Fine,' he says, 'it looks worse than it is.'

We chat for a couple of minutes but he's not able to maintain the conversation and neither am I. I am devastated to see him in such pain, with this tube coming out of him. I am struggling to get my head around this. Hopefully that is the worst of it over now. The doctors have said it will take him three days to come around properly. If he heals well he could be out in five. There's comfort for everyone in that.

He soon needs to sleep, so we are forced to leave him. We stop for a hot chocolate downstairs before we go. A sugar boost is needed. There's such a sense of uncertainty about all this. So far there's been little talk of further treatment. The words 'lung' and 'cancer' have also faded into the background. Maybe they're not sure that's what it is any more. Or perhaps it's not as bad as they think and they are re-evaluating their next move. Perhaps this procedure was all he needed.

JULY–AUGUST 2013

4

MAKING A PLAN

It's been a few weeks now since Dad's surgery and he's recovering well. They removed the tube from his side the day after the procedure, as they were pleased it was a success. He was released on day five, as expected, and was only too delighted to get home. His breathing seems normal again, which means his lung is not refilling with fluid. Fantastic. His wounds are still healing and Mum has been over to his apartment, dressing and changing the bandages twice daily for him.

These past few weeks have been unexpectedly and surprisingly lovely. Mum and Dad seem to have really reconnected. From the outside looking in I can see Mum is still trying to figure out her *exact* or *right* place in all of this. Maybe there is no *exact* or *right* place. Maybe it's just about taking each day as it comes and doing what feels right. It appears, though, that she's definitely made the decision to stand beside him through all of this. I am both moved and grateful. It's a scary time for everyone and having Mum by all our sides is an immeasurable weight off our shoulders.

Normality has resumed in other areas. Dad is back playing the guitar in The Hot Spot, the local café and music venue in Greystones, run by a wonderful lady called Ailbhe, where people come to play, sing and jam together. Dad has also been expressing aspirations to get back to his boxing. We all just ignored these comments. He knows our feelings on the matter. Why can't he just join a nice safe walking club, or take up aqua aerobics or something? Aside from that, the sense of normality in all this is uplifting.

Tomorrow we have a meeting with the oncologist. This is the meeting we've been waiting for. All the tests have been done, the Talc Pleurodesis has been done and recovery from that is well underway. Now we need to know what treatment is going to help Dad get better. Nothing can be done until his wounds from the surgery have healed completely, but they are healing nicely, which we take as a good sign.

Whatever happens tomorrow we will deal with it. Should the prognosis be less positive than we want, or should the suggested treatment be as aggressive as last time, we will still get him through it.

This man is going nowhere.

**

I'm not there for the news.

After waiting with Dad, Mum and Ciara outside the oncologist's office in St Vincent's for three hours, I had to leave and go back to work. They were in decent form when I left, despite the wait and our reasons for being there. Dad's stitches have healed and he looks completely healthy again, so it's strange to be here waiting for a plan going forward – which will include chemo, no doubt. I'm just hoping it won't be too aggressive.

I finish up my day in the studio at six o'clock. I haven't spoken to anyone since leaving the hospital. No news is good news, I think. I'm due to meet them in a local Italian restaurant we like to frequent and will get the gist of the meeting then.

They are already there when I arrive. I sit down beside Dad, facing Mum and Ciara. Stephen has to work late and I'm not sure if anyone has spoken to him yet. It only takes me a second to read Ciara's body language: uptight with a lack of eye contact.

Shit. Whatever they have to say it is definitely negative.

I just don't want to hear more bad news right now. And so I don't ask how they got on in the hospital. I'm not ready. I start to blabber on about my day, talking nonsense. It's funny, I feel like an outsider sitting at the table. Like they're all part of some secret group to which I don't have membership. But I want to stay in my ignorance and feel like an alien for just a little longer. So the blabbering continues until the waiter comes to take our order and cuts me off.

When the waiter leaves silence settles on the table.

Shit.

Dad starts. 'So we weren't waiting that long after you left today. I'd say maybe another half an hour.'

'Oh, that's great,' I reply.

'We had a good chat with the oncologist and discussed everything. To be honest with you there's no other way to look at this, honey. It just isn't good news.'

'Okay. Sorry. But that sentence has been bandied around constantly for the last month. Like, how bad is "not good"?'

'Well, it turns out the tumour has grown right through my lung,' he says, shifting slightly in his seat. 'This basically means that the cancer cells are no longer contained in my lung.' He makes eye contact with Mum as he continues. 'They have escaped through the breach into the rest of my body. This, unfortunately, leaves no option of operating and radiotherapy won't work because it's not specific to one area any more.'

Right. Distressing information overload. I can feel the tears welling up in my eyes. I start massaging the lump in my throat. It's so sore and tight. I look at Mum and Ciara. It must have been really hard for them to hear this news directly. I imagine them in the room earlier, all three of them getting this news, and it makes me even sadder.

'So you do chemo then, yeah?'

'Yes, I will do chemo every month and that will buy me some time.'

Time? What is he on about – time? Time. What? That's a ridiculous comment to make.

'There are also other things we can do and I fully intend to do them, so all is not lost. There is a decompression chamber that I am going to try. Ciara has already been looking into the benefits of that and is doing great research there. I am going big into the greens and will juice daily. I am going to cut out any sugar and crap food from my diet to keep it out of an acidic state. They say that sugar is a major contributing factor to cancer. There's lots there to look at.'

'Okay,' I whisper, still fighting the lump in my throat. 'Well, that's good.' Finally some sort of good news or at least something proactive we can do to assist in driving us forward to our main goal: Dad's survival.

'You need to know though, hun, the outcome is not going to change much here but I am going to give it all I've got, to get as long as I can with you guys. They're saying I've got about eight to ten months.'

I feel like a deer caught in headlights. I'm trying to think of positive things to say. I can't. I'm all out. My throat is screaming with the pressure of holding back. I cannot accept this.

'Unfortunately there just isn't a cure,' he continues. 'It's all about getting as much time as we can. The cells are everywhere now and you need to understand that.'

I can't see now. I have a wall of tears in my eyes. Like a dam overflowing, the tears spill out and stream down my face. *Oh, sweet Jesus.* I need to go to the bathroom; I cannot do this here. I drop my head and look down, trying to let the one side of longer hair that I have cover what it can of my face. It's at times like this that I wish I still had long hair. I keep my mouth shut; I have no idea what might come out if I try to utter a single word.

Keeping my head down, I remove my napkin from my lap, stand up and head straight for the bathroom. *This cannot be. This cannot be.* I push the door open and hold on to the bathroom wall with one hand for support, the other holding my stomach. I just stand there, tears streaming. I feel like I need to wail but I can't. In fact, no noise comes out at all. I am nearly retching I am crying so hard, but still there is no noise.

Eventually I stop crying and manage to catch my breath. I look up and stare at myself in the mirror. I've never seen my face look so devastated. My dad cannot die. My dad *cannot* die. Jesus, even these words in the same sentence are too much. Another round of convulsions starts. I know I'm thirty but I feel too young to lose my dad. He'll never get to meet my kids, if I ever have them. Okay, this is not an option. This just cannot happen.

Mum walks in. With all these thoughts in my head I look up at her as if to say, 'What the fuck is actually happening here?'

'I know, Lisa, it's so hard to hear that. We went into the little chapel in St Vincent's after we got the news and had a cry. It is just so hard to believe this is happening.'

Hard? Understatement of the year.

I can feel the anger starting now. This is a load of bollocks. There's no way this is going to happen. Not on my watch. Absolutely not. I need to get in there and speak to that oncologist myself. There absolutely, positively has to be more that can be done. Anyway, what are they doing telling the man that there's not much to be done? It's like the power of suggestion. He'll have himself dead and buried by next week with that kind of medical attitude. We need to work on his mental state now to make sure he does not believe this crap. Stupid doctors. Have they done all they can, *really*? I bet you they haven't. Oh, the anger is there, all right. I actually want to knock the head off that oncologist right now.

Mum gets some toilet roll and hands it to me. I badly need it. I'm a complete mess and a far cry from presentable.

I'm not a big fan of people seeing me cry. In fact, I'm not a big fan of people seeing me be anything less than okay. This is especially the case in front of people I don't know. I'm only comfortable with people very close seeing me break down; it's only with them that I can really open up. My dad is at the very top of the list of people I would go to for that sort of release. He always slags me when I say, 'I'm fine.'

'Fine?' he'd say. 'You know what that stands for? Fucked up, Insecure, Neurotic and Emotional. Oh yeah, you're fine alright!'

'Ha ha, Dad,' I'd reply, laughing along with him.

'It is okay to be vulnerable, Lisa,' he'd add, in all seriousness.

I'll get there one day, maybe, but for now this emotional meltdown can stay in the bathroom.

It suddenly comes to my attention that Mum had to hear this news earlier.

'You okay?' I ask.

'Yeah, I'm all right. It's going to be a tough road ahead of us, though.'

Her comment forces me to consider what now lies ahead of us. I hadn't given that any thought. I reach ahead in time for a second but quickly snap myself back, my head about to explode. No. That's not a good idea for me. I instinctively know I will have to take each day as it comes from now on. Dealing only with whatever happens in one day. I will not be able to cope if I look too far ahead.

We hug and ready ourselves to rejoin Ciara and Dad. This cancer has a seriously strong-minded family on its ass, and I'm convinced there's more we can do. If anyone can beat the odds it's Gerry Collins and, with the weight of the Collins family behind him, he has every chance.

***

I'm due to meet Dad for a catch-up in a coffee shop in Delgany. The last few weeks since his sentence was delivered have been really busy. It feels like cancer has quickly invaded every conscious thought. There is very little else any more; almost no room at all for general day-to-day thoughts. It's just cancer, research and our mission to beat it.

The 'go to' treatment for this is obviously chemo, but we are also researching any other options we can try in conjunction with that, and we fully intend to throw everything we can at this that has a chance of helping Dad. The news has spread further afield now, from family to friends to my clients. As a result, a lot of information is coming at us and I am also proactively seeking it in any way I can. There's lots of talk about things that can help cure cancer, so it's hard to know what to focus on first, and we have no idea if any of it works, but we are prepared to try everything. One or all of these alternative cures is bound to make a difference, right?

I meet Dad upstairs and we talk about what he's doing. He's started back boxing – training lightly, he says, and playing loads of guitar. He's also due to start chemo soon, which he is not looking forward to.

After our coffee, we head to the health shop downstairs to tackle the first thing on our mission list – improving his diet. We have continuously heard in recent weeks about how good nutrition is so important for people living with cancer, particularly beans, lentils and vegetables.

We soon get chatting to the woman who runs the place, who, as it turns out, had cancer herself a few years ago. Honestly, the more we talk to people the less surprised I am when they say they've had cancer. At this point it seems like there are fewer people who haven't had cancer! This lady is a mine of information. She claims she healed herself without chemo, simply by changing her diet from a state of acidic to alkaline.

'Sorry, hang on a second!' I cry as I grapple through my bag for my phone and quickly open up my notes app. 'Okay, go on, you were saying. Actually, no, sorry, can you start again? I forgot what you were saying about sugar.' I am not missing a thing.

The conversation goes on for an hour. It was like a crash course in all things healthy. My overall understanding of her model is that sugary foods, beige foods like pasta, bread, pizzas, etc., as well as wines, beers, chocolate (Dad's favourite thing) and pretty much anything food-related that can bring you pleasure, are out. She believes that they all bring your body out of a state of alkaline and into a state of acidic, which she says is a stomping ground for cancerous cells. This is something we've heard before from other people.

I'm no expert, but her advice makes me feel really hopeful. This is something we can do and if it helps that'd be amazing. However, although Dad and I are equally enthused about saving his life, I now sense another burning issue. On a daily basis, what will be the cost to his happiness of this voyage towards a strictly green diet? It may seem like a trivial concern – in many ways it is – but when a man is suffering from lung cancer and his appetite is a challenge on a good day, how likely is he, really, to sit down to a bowl of alfalfa and lentils and still be happy? This could be a tall order. But, true to the man he is, he will go to any lengths to succeed in what he sets his mind to. So off we go back to the car, slightly bamboozled, with two bags full of wheatgrass seeds to be planted (we now need to go and buy compost and trays), a ridiculous amount of green vegetables, most of which I don't know the names of, and a cookbook full of recipes for an alkaline diet. At least we're doing something, right?

So that's his diet covered.

Our next target is the oxygen chamber. Let's discuss.

Firstly, this is not a proven treatment for cancer. Unfortunately. However, further to Ciara's countless hours of research, she has argued that it's definitely worth a shot. What the oxygen chambers are said to do is enhance the body's natural healing process, working on the basis that inhalation of pure oxygen assists our red blood cells to deliver better oxygenated blood to areas of need in the body. So, with this in mind, Ciara reasons that it has the potential to assist any damaged tissue within Dad's body, thereby aiding recovery where possible. It makes sense to me. He's booked in for next week, so we'll see then how he gets on. Ciara is going in with him.

The next thing to be considered is hemp oil. Something about this came up in my news feed last night. In it I read that hemp oil was basically marijuana in liquid form, but without the chemical that makes you high. The article urged that people who had cancer should start taking this straight away, as it apparently helps ease the effects of chemo and could even save lives.

Now, when I say I spent the next few hours researching this, I mean I was up until 3 a.m. that night, trawling through medical marijuana websites, hemp oil cures cancer websites, the different ways in which one can smoke, ingest, inject and drink the stuff, even going so far as to search websites on how to import or smuggle this illegal drug into Ireland. It was hard to know what information and which studies were legitimate, because there are so many sites with such different information, but what I did read really made me wonder: if it truly could heal our bodies, though I'm still not exactly sure how it's supposed to do that, would it not be worth a try?

In the clear light of the following day, I'm feeling empowered. With time not being in our favour, it's an exhausting rush to find out everything and get all the things he needs *right now*. The sheer terror of finding a cure weeks after he dies is too much.

As a result, it appears my next move may be to attempt to import an illegal substance into the country.

The lengths we consider going to for the ones we love!

5

SO IT BEGINS

In between all the alternative cure searching, Dad's first chemo is upon us before we know it. I'm uneasy thinking of what lies ahead. In many ways, the thought of him doing chemo last time was easier for us. We were all going in blind and had no idea what he was facing into.

This time we do.

It reminds me – though obviously this is no comparison – of a bus journey I did in Laos from Luang Prabang to Vang Vieng in my early twenties. It was hands down the most terrifying journey I have ever taken. The journey took seven hours, the majority of it down a steep, treacherous mountain in the pitch black. The bus had to go fast so bandits wouldn't ambush it and rob the passengers, and it could only stop at designated rest areas, of which there were few. It went down from such a height at such a speed that most of the passengers, including myself, had to vomit into plastic bags due to altitude and motion sickness. Had this bus veered even slightly off its track it would have gone over the mountainside, which would have meant certain death for everyone on board. I took that bus journey because I had no idea of what was ahead of me, and even if someone told me that my life now depended on my repeating that journey, I am not sure I would do it.

I do not voice these thoughts to Dad, obviously, but they are there. I know he has no choice and I'm hopeful that it will buy him more time, as they're claiming. The doctors also say that it won't be as bad this time. His dosage is lower. He'll only be doing four hours of chemo one day a week every two weeks, whereas last time he did courses of twenty-four hours, five days a week every three weeks.

Mum is bringing him in today for his first round. Thank God for her. If she wasn't here I really don't know what Stephen, Ciara and I would do. The worry alone of it all takes a toll and there's also a lot of medical information to take in. We'd be lost without her. Unfortunately I have to work, so can't go with them, but I will follow in an hour or two.

I give him a quick buzz when he's on the way in. 'Dad, you all set?'

'Sure am. Have you many clients in today?'

Honestly. He's sincerely more interested in talking about my business than he is about his appointment.

'Loads in today; it's all good.' *Anyway.* 'How are you feeling about heading in, Dad? You've got Florence Nightingale beside you so you should be grand.'

'Absolutely. I'm in great hands. I'm all psyched up and ready to kick some cancer ass.'

He sounds determined.

'Great stuff, Dad, I've just a few more clients here, then I'll follow you guys in.'

'Okay, love, see you then.'

***

A while later, I head to St Vincent's. As I drive, I think about where I'm going to park. It costs a small fortune to park in the hospital car park. Then I feel a sudden tinge of guilt at the fact that I'm thinking about the cost of such things at a time like this. It's weird the things I feel bad about these days. I find it hard to allow myself to laugh too much, or enjoy anything too much right now. Dad's entire life has literally stopped in its tracks. Everything that was once certain for him is certain no longer. Everything he had envisioned for the future is no longer a given. Nothing is as it was.

That's the thing I've noticed about cancer. You try not to let it change anything, but it does. It changes everything. Including your priorities. This, I find, is what distresses me the most. I am now forced into a situation full of conflicting priorities. On one hand, I have a member of my family who is very sick and needs looking after. All I want to do is be there to help him and understand every doctor's report and find any cure or solution of which we might avail ourselves. On the other hand, I have a life full of responsibilities that need to be tended to – even though these commitments, which I once deemed hugely important in my life, seem almost trivial now. I am constantly fighting the gravitational pull of these responsibilities that continue to drag me forward in my own life, so I can stop and stand still with

Dad. But it just doesn't work; at times, I can't stop life from pulling me on, away from him.

I refocus as I arrive at St Vincent's. I've never been to the Oncology Day Centre before, so I'm unsure which way to go. I stop and ask a member of staff as I walk into the reception area. It's not far, I'm told, and follow their directions right and then down to the end of the building.

I have butterflies in my stomach by the time I reach the day ward. I notice how bright and clean it is. Even though it's a sterile environment it feels warm, which is comforting. I see nurses with friendly faces, which is also comforting. I turn the corner and see a row of chemo chairs along a big wall in the chemo ward. It's quite an open-plan ward, with curtains pushed back to their starting positions. Privacy for this treatment, it seems, isn't completely necessary. I immediately see Dad in the last one, with Mum beside him in a regular chair. I also see the drip leading into his right arm. My stomach lurches. I just cannot get my head around the idea of voluntarily pumping this poison into him. *This is a good thing, Lisa*, I remind myself. *This is a good thing.*

'Hey guys. How are you doing, Dad? You're looking good, anyway.'

A throwaway compliment is never wasted in situations like this.

He laughs. 'Wouldn't expect anything less!'

'Did they find a vein okay?'

I only know to ask this question from experience. At times, previously, it was a tough slog trying to find a good vein.

'They did and everything's fine. I just need to sit here for three more hours and then I should be good to go.'

'Great stuff,' I say.

I grab a vacant stool and pull it over beside them. As I sit down I notice Dad looks like he's had two weeks in Spain since I saw him a couple of days ago. This, I also know from experience, is from the steroids. They make his skin brown. He has to take them for three days before the chemo and two days after, so his body can handle it. I'm not entirely sure how they help or why they make him look tanned, but they do. The 'tanned look' usually disappears after a week or so, but he's left quite bloated after them. He hates that.

'Not a good look,' he'd say. 'I'm far too good-looking to don the bloated look.' He'd laugh, but he means it. 'At least I'll make a good-looking corpse' is another joke he likes to make and 'definitely an open casket for me'. The funny thing is those are jokes he made even when he wasn't sick. Now that he is sick, we still hear them. You can't help but laugh in response.

We sit and chat and they give me updates on how great the nurses are here. I think he may have charmed them already, as a couple of them have been over fussing since I've been here, all of ten minutes. He's singing their praises, which is nice to hear. At least he feels he is in good hands.

I look around and feel a strong jolt of shock. There are so many people here. What is our world coming to? I notice one young guy in particular. My age, I'd say, or maybe a year or two older. Early thirties, anyway. He's two chairs down from Dad. He's a good-looking guy, very tall, with brown eyes and dark hair. Although he has his head shaved quite tightly, I can see that his hair is falling out as the stubble is patchy. I imagine his natural skin shade to be quite sallow but he looks extremely pale and tired, leaving him looking gaunt and low in vitality. As he sits there with the drip in his right arm, he's reading some sort of sports magazine. He senses me staring and lifts his head. I get a bit of a fright but I nod and give him a half smile. He half-smiles in return and then puts his head back down to continue reading.

Will he be okay? Surely he will. Right? I mean, if it's too early for my dad to go, by God it has to be too early for this poor lad. My mind can't help but wonder how this awful disease has affected his life. Has he had to stop working? What do people in his work think about all this? Might he be self-employed too? Has anyone secretly thought he brought it on himself by his lifestyle choices? Perhaps their own mortality and poor life habits have been highlighted to them by the sheer fact that this young guy now has cancer. Has it given them perspective? Is he as blessed with his family as we are with ours? I hope they are minding him. There is no one with him right now but that's not to say they haven't just nipped out.

Watching him sit there on his own, looking so unwell, makes me think. People who are sick need people who are well to mind them – that's just the way of it. It's too tough otherwise. Sick people have no energy to cook or clean or change sheets. They don't have the energy to run to the shops and get what they need for the week ahead. They sometimes don't even have the energy to talk. I look back at Dad. He's chatting to Mum about going for a walk next weekend. He likes to have things to look forward to. I hope he'll be well enough to go on this walk.

The three hours pass and he's done. The nurse takes the drip out and Dad appears fine. Mum and I take our time leaving the hospital. The magnitude of Dad having just finished his first chemo session weighs heavily on me as I walk along the corridor, linked arm in arm with Mum. Dad, on the other hand, has speed-walked up the corridor ahead of us and has already reached the door. He waves at us to hurry. When we reach him, he tells us that he wants the keys from Mum. He insists that he is fine to drive. Mum reluctantly gives him the keys. She has no choice, really. When Dad decides he is doing something, he does it.

I drive behind them the whole way home and wave to them as I take the homeward-bound turn off into Charlesland. Mum is bringing Dad home to his apartment and getting him sorted. He apparently wants to go play some guitar with John. He's manic from the steroids – a common side effect – so during these times we just have to go with him while continuously reminding him to take it as easy as he can.

Kat greets me as I walk into my apartment. She has dinner made. Excellent. It's only now that I realise how hungry I am. Her friend, Michelle, is here and they are having wine in the kitchen. Michelle is a lovely girl. Her mum died of cancer a good few years ago, when she was in her early teens. Tragic as her story is, it gives me hope. Seeing her functioning like a proper human after such a massive loss makes me think that I just might make it too, if I am faced with the same loss.

For a time I stand and talk with the girls – until, that is, I feel a sudden surge of emotion inside me. I can't quite listen to anything they're saying; I keep seeing the chemo going into Dad's arm.

I go to the bathroom and let the tears out. I have already started to look at them as being like a release valve. When the valve is full, it needs to be released. That's just the way it is.

My phone rings in my bag. I look. It's Dad.

'Hiya, hun, you doing okay?'

'Hey, Dad, yeah, I'm grand. Kat has some dinner on so we're going to sit down and have that in a few minutes.'

'You've been crying,' he says. *How does he do that?* 'Listen, I know this is hard, Lisa. I know going into hospital and seeing me in there again today must be really difficult. Just remember that this is going to buy me more time, so this really is a good thing.'

'Dad! It's going to do more than that, don't say things like that.'

'I know, I know. I'm not saying anything, hun. It's such a tough time for everyone right now but we will get through it together. Don't worry about crying; get the tears out. I am going to give this everything I've got. Honestly, I feel fine after today. John's just left after playing a few tunes, so it's all good.'

Well, that's good, I suppose. He does sound in good spirits.

'Get some sleep and let's meet for coffee tomorrow,' he says in a calming voice.

Lovely. That's grand. I'll see him tomorrow.

We say goodnight and I get into bed early. Kat's so good and brings me up dinner in bed. It's still bright out but I close the curtains, get the laptop out, watch an episode of *Orange is the new Black* and try to eat my dinner.

SEPTEMBER–OCTOBER 2013

6

LIFE ACCORDING
TO CHEMO

Over the last eight weeks, since that initial round of chemo, Dad has had three more rounds of chemo, which now brings him up to a total of four sessions.

Today I expect he'll be tired. He's been very down the last few days and hasn't wanted many visitors. He's been responding to the odd few texts here and there, but we're worried. He sits in his chair a lot these days. Depending on where he is in his chemo cycle, he's either too ill and weak, or recovering and too exhausted to do much.

He was fine after the first one. It seemed barely to affect him. The second chemo was pretty much the same, although he crashed a bit from the steroids and got a bit low in himself for a few days. But he went boxing and continued to work out and that helped bring him back up.

The second one was a gentle reminder of what was ahead, though, because it was then he started to address the problem of what he was going to do when he was too sick to work. As we all know, the self-employed can't get sick. At the very beginning of all this, Dad couldn't find the time to be even *mildly* unwell or miss a business meeting; now, his cares from before are not even *remotely* important. He has been forced to change his priorities completely. His only priority now is survival. Any excess or unnecessary stress is to be removed immediately from his life, or a plan put in place to address it and relieve it.

His third and fourth chemo sessions were much harder on his body. He needed more days to recover, which left fewer days where he was well enough to go out or go boxing. God knows he tried. The lack of exercise is affecting him mentally. The last few weeks have undoubtedly been the toughest yet. He puts on a brave face, but he is in pain a lot of the time now. I often see him grabbing or holding his left side, which is a painful reminder of the tumour that is inside him. I constantly stare at his left side when he's not looking, willing the tumour away.

He rings me mid-morning, asking that I bring him a copy of *The Irish Times*. I call over in the hope of spending some time with him, though I suspect it'll be a short visit. I grab some chocolate, too, at the shop. Just in case he's able. Fuck the diet.

When I arrive to his place I see that he's left the door open. I walk straight into the sitting room. He's sitting in his chair, looking out the window. He looks pale and distraught. The look on his face strikes me hard. I don't say a word. Something is going on. He turns his head fully and looks directly at me. I can see his face starting to crumble. It's a look that is not altogether familiar yet I know I've seen it once before.

He needs to let all this out.

I rush to him. He's not well enough to stand. I sit on the side arm of his chair and hug him tightly as he bursts into tears. 'I'm so sorry!' he cries and holds onto my arm. 'I'm so sorry!'

I shake my head, unable to speak, to say, 'You've nothing to be sorry about.'

I can sense why he's crying, though. His apologies are full of pain and despair. He knows that he cannot take back all those cigarettes smoked. He cannot go back and undo all his past wrongs.

I scramble for words to help ease his pain but I just don't know what to say. The enormity of the situation is beyond me. So I hug him tighter.

'I'm so sorry I won't be here for you guys!' he mourns as he cries into his hands.

'Dad!' I cry, my arm still around him. 'This is not your fault. This is just a shit hand that's been dealt and is *so fucking shit* it's unbelievable.'

He hates me cursing but, in this case, I feel it is totally necessary to emphasise my point.

In an effort to further comfort him I lean my forehead against the side of his head. As I do so I am struck by how soft his hair is and am instantly hit with a memory of Gang Gang. The memory is of me as a little girl and it starts playing like a movie in front of my eyes. I'm sitting on the side arm of my grandad's chair, brushing his soft grey hair with my little blue brush. Dad, in *his* thirties, is standing there talking to his dad about work and some deal he was working on. I can clearly remember how contented I felt as I sat there, brushing Grandad's hair and just being with them.

And now, here I sit, on the side arm of my dad's chair, holding him in a vulnerable moment as he's faced with his own mortality. He will take the journey next, after his own father, as I will take it after him. And so on. The cycle of life.

Something that's never occurred to me before is now very clear. This is a lonely path that no one can protect us from. We must all face our own final journey alone.

It must be so frightening.

He continues to cry and I continue to hold him. My arm feels so small around his broad shoulders but I hold on tight. As the tears subside, I pull myself up and get him some tissues from the bathroom.

When I return there's a lift in the air. The moment is over. I hand him some tissues.

'Thanks,' he says, taking them. He leans back into his chair as he dries his eyes.

'Oh, Dad. You poor thing. Are you okay?'

'Yeah, honey, thanks for that.' He looks wrecked. 'That's been coming for a couple of months, I think. I just feel so bad at the moment.'

This was definitely needed. We've been so focused on fighting the cancer with such relentless determination that it has allowed little room for Dad to feel the inevitable and natural emotions of what he's going through.

'Would you like some tea?' I offer. Tea always makes things better.

'A glass of water would be great, thanks.'

I pass him the newspaper before I head to the kitchen. I'm not gone long but he's fast asleep when I return. I put a blanket over him and put the TV on quietly. He's got tinnitus from the chemo so he can't hear it. I sit and stare at it. Completely stunned by the beautiful, raw moment I got to share with him, I'm just content to be here with him. Even when he's asleep.

Last week, John did something that, I thought, was the essence of a true friend. He unexpectedly arrived over to Dad's place armed with three pots, three plants, a big bag of soil and a bucket of window-cleaning products.

'Right, Gerry,' he declared. 'You may not be able to go outside as much at the moment so we better make sure you can see the outside perfectly! You sit right there and watch me wash your windows. This is not something you will see very often, Gerry Collins, so enjoy it! Not only that, I am going to pot you some plants. Yes, you heard me, Gerry, plants, to create some feng shui. This should help bring the energy levels up.'

John has since laughed if off, making light of it, but the meaning behind it is undiluted: it is an act of pure love for a friend.

Needless to say Dad sat and watched and smiled. He didn't have the energy to say much but he was utterly moved.

***

Two days after the fifth chemo session, Mum calls and asks me to pick up some Motilium ASAP and bring it to Dad's place. She sounds panicked on the phone so I don't waste any time.

When I arrive at the apartment Dad is sitting in his chair as usual. As I walk in Mum catches my eye. She looks worried.

I walk towards Dad to say hi and to give him his Motilium. He looks extremely pale and like he's lost a stone overnight. As I near him, he immediately puts one hand over his nose and mouth. Looking completely horrified, he throws his other hand towards me to push me away.

'Lisa, get out!' he shouts.

I stop dead in my tracks, my hand still holding the Motilium out towards him.

'Jesus, Lisa, I can't bear it. You'll have to get out.'

There is sheer panic in his voice. I don't think I've ever seen him freak out like this and I have no idea why. I look at Mum standing there. She looks as shocked as I feel.

Suddenly Dad leans over the chair and starts aggressively retching. Mum runs and grabs a basin from under the sink and puts it on the floor under him and rubs his back. He is retching hard and fast now. I can see the blood vessels on the side of his temples. Oh my God, this is obviously because of me, somehow. I must have done something. I just don't know what.

Dad can't speak but he looks up for a second and there are tears in his eyes, his face is red and purple from the pressure and he's now urgently pointing towards the door for me to go.

'Oh my God, Dad, are you okay?'

Horrified, I start to back up towards the sitting-room door. I throw the Motilium on the table and turn on my heels and run towards the front door, tears streaming down my face.

Just as I pull the front door open, I hear Dad shout, 'Lisa!

I'm sorry. Hang on!' His voice is strained and forced because of the retching.

I stop. I can hear him trying to catch his breath.

'It's your perfume, Lisa. It's the chemo. It makes your perfume smell like lead. I can taste it, it's so strong. I'm sorry. Just wait there for a minute.'

But I'm not wearing any perfume. I know his sense of smell is heightened from the chemo. I'm so careful not to wear any perfume around him. I am one hundred per cent sure.

Mum has come out to me now. She gives me a big hug and I bawl into her arms.

'I'm not wearing any perfume,' I say. 'I swear to God I'm not. I know better than that.'

Something has obviously set him off big time, but what?

'Can you smell me?' I ask. She is sniffing all around me now. I twirl.

'No, but I can get a very, *very*, faint smell of something from the back of you, I think.'

Eh what? The back of me? What on earth can that be? Then it hits me.

'Oh my God. My deodorant!' I exclaim. I definitely put some on this morning. 'I didn't even think.'

'That's what it is,' Mum nods. 'It's the aluminium salts in the deodorant.'

Mum raises her voice so Dad can hear. 'Gerry, it's her deodorant. It's the aluminium salts reacting with the chemo.'

'I'm so sorry, honey. You'll have to go,' Dad calls out weakly. His retching has eased off now, thankfully. 'Thank you for the tablets. I guess it's just another thing we need to watch out for. I hope you're okay. I'll give you a buzz later.'

I give Mum a hug and shout to Dad that I'm fine and sorry and I hope he's okay. I leave the apartment, the adrenaline still pumping around my body. I've never had a fright like that before, ever.

God, I hate chemo.

7

REFLECTION

In calm moments between the chemo cycles I find myself reflecting a lot. I don't know what's ahead of me but I do know I need to be at my fittest emotionally, mentally and spiritually to cope. What we are dealing with is tough stuff.

When it was confirmed that Dad had terminal lung cancer I wanted to talk to anyone who'd listen about this terrible news that had been thrust upon my dad, my family and, essentially, me. There are two main reasons for this. One, I'm an emotional person and I like to talk through things. And two, I was trying to gather useful information to include in our mission to help Dad.

It's human nature for people to want to share similar experiences with each other. It's called identification. There's a sense of support and understanding for us when we can relate to one another and with that comes a feeling of security in knowing you are not alone. I have had the honour of having some truly wonderful conversations with people sharing their own cancer stories and how they managed it all. Some have been incredibly helpful.

There's another reason we like to talk: knowledge. Those people who have previously walked down this unknown and frightening road may have some invaluable information to impart to us. Perhaps we can avoid the mistakes they made. Perhaps we can succeed where they or their loved ones didn't.

I had a good chat recently with a client of mine, Joy, whose name reflects her in every way. She had not only lost her dad but also her mum when she was in her twenties. When I hear things like that it really hammers home just how resilient we humans can actually be. I just don't think I'd have survived that blow. She gifted me with three essential pieces of information, which I wrote down after she left:

1. Get loads of footage of your dad. Film anything and everything. It doesn't matter what he's doing – record it. Just make sure to record his voice. You will forever be glad you can hear his voice, especially when you're older.

2. Have the conversations you want to have *early*. Don't leave them until *later*. People think to have 'those' conversations too late. He'll be too physically sick then and won't be able for them.

3. *Never* fight with your family during this time. Emotions are heightened beyond a point you may have never experienced before. Things will be said out of rage, sadness, grief, etc. If someone says something that offends you say absolutely nothing. Let the dust settle and tend to it later. It's at times like this and after funerals that family feuds can happen, so fix any rifts immediately.

Her words ring in my ears daily. In fact, I've already taken her first point on board. I feel like a sneaky paparazzo half the time, just missing my sunglasses and hat. I try to be subtle with the camera but I get the feeling I may be making him feel weird, under the circumstances. Nevertheless, I shall continue.

This whole period is a massive learning curve for everyone in the family. Each person is trying to navigate their way through it, as best they can. As I watch each member of my family, it strikes me how differently we are all dealing with this. But we have the right to deal with it in our own way. It's too easy to get pissed off with other family members who 'should be doing more', or 'shouldn't have said that', 'should have spoken up' or 'didn't help out with that situation'. The list goes on. You just have to believe that people are doing their best. Otherwise the anger – just or unjust – will eat you up.

Denial also has a big part to play in this process. I used to think denial was a choice. That a person chose to ignore a situation, or look the other way, because it's easier than having to face it – or worse, actually having to do something about it. I used to think it was weak and it was an excuse. But I now understand that denial is actually a form of protection. Our human minds can only process or handle so much at one time. You never know what someone is dealing with at any given time in his or her life, or what they're contending with in their minds. Then throw sickness, chemo, hospital appointments and a real threat of death into the mix. It's a lot. People go into denial because their autopilot/subconscious is protecting them. There's a saying, 'Denial is not just a river in Egypt.' Well, I have a feeling we all, at different times, dip into that big fat stream of relief, looking to cool down when the heat gets too much.

Realising that I am already struggling with all this, and in an effort to arm myself for what's ahead, I have decided to do some psychotherapy. If something is, in fact, going to happen to Dad, then I need to be the strongest I have ever been in my life. I need any unresolved issues sorted. Any potential cracks filled. I am going to need help dealing with the few months ahead because when I'm not splashing around in Egypt, my brain is drip-feeding me heavy doses of reality. Some days I can deal with the sucker punches and other days it feels like I have been physically hit by a freight train. I have found this amazing woman in Killiney – I've only been twice so far but I feel like she is going to be my lifeline. From here on I'm just going to do what I can do. Control what I can control. I'll continue researching cures, going to hospital appointments, getting stuff in the pharmacy and just generally being where I'm needed.

I've noticed at this point that I'm starting to veer further away from having 'cancer conversations' with people. I'm not as able for them any more. It seems the past pains of others are now a little too close to my current living reality – especially those stories that do not have a happy ending.

Yesterday I popped into my mum's for a quick cuppa. Her friend Breda was there, whom I hadn't seen in quite a while. Naturally, as it does now, the conversation veered towards this cancer business. Then she started to recount the story of her own father and his battle with bowel cancer over seven years ago. As I listened to her devastating story, a sense of alarm started to rise. I knew where this story was going. Her dad died. There was no happy ending. As she continued, I just wanted to bolt for the door.

'So, unfortunately, towards the end they couldn't find any veins in his arms or hands and they had to put the drip in his feet,' she said at one point.

Oh God, I thought. They do tend to struggle to find a vein in Dad's arms. Would he now be faced with the same fate?

It's too frightening to hear these stories now. We're too far down the rabbit hole. One positive I did take from this episode was that she herself appeared to have detached from her own story. She has tapped out of the rawness in which she once lived. She, for the most part, appears to have 'moved on'.

This I will hold on to for later.

For now, between all the madness, I am trying to quietly build myself up from the inside out. I have no idea as to what's ahead and it terrifies me. My stomach is in turmoil a lot of the time, so I'm finding it hard to eat. As a result, I'm also trying to nourish myself from the outside in.

I'm going over to Dad's tomorrow to watch *Love/Hate*. I couldn't think of a better way to spend a Sunday evening.

I'm holding on to as much 'normal' as possible.

***

After that last chemo Dad has decided to take a break from it and give his body a chance to recover. The irony of taking a break from the very thing that's meant to be saving you so that you can recover is not lost on me. I'm glad, to be honest. It was getting too aggressive.

I have this constant nagging pain in my chest at the moment; it's not really bad but it's always there. I rest a hot water bottle on it at night to help me sleep. I find it helps.

Work is on my mind a lot. I've only had to reschedule a couple of clients so far and they were so accommodating. However, last week, when I unexpectedly had to change an appointment, the client couldn't reschedule and I was forced to organise it so that she went to someone else. It was a small thing but it really added to my stress levels. I'm worried about how I am going to manage all this. I know I will be there for my dad and family, no question, but who will be there for my clients?

It's just me, after all. If I'm not there, I'm not making money. How is that going to pan out when my dad is dying? After he dies? I can't even imagine the pain I will be in. How do people do this? I honestly do not think I will survive if he dies. Never mind work. And I'll have to go back straight away because it's just me there to bring an income in.

Breathe, Lisa.

One day, I arrange to meet Dad for a coffee between clients, to shoot the breeze and have the chats, as we do. The venue for our meeting is a gorgeous café in the Arboretum Garden Centre in Kilquade. It almost looks like a large greenhouse and is surrounded by every type of plant you can imagine, with a beautiful waterfall behind it. I had my thirtieth there last May actually. We had the whole place to ourselves. It wasn't a big affair but it was perfect. It was the happiest evening of my life.

I just felt on top of the world with all my closest family and friends in a wonderful place surrounded by beauty and nature. Dad gave such a lovely speech that night. I'll never forget it.

I arrive before him and get a table beside the window. He arrives only a few minutes after me. It's a breath of fresh air to see him out and about again. The difference in him without the chemo is unbelievable. He's in great form. I have already ordered us tea and no doubt he will have some sort of cake. He has such a sweet tooth. He's trying his best to stay away from sugar as part of this new alkaline diet, but it's very difficult for him. I don't judge when I see him eat some chocolate or biscuits. I feel for the man. His taste buds were badly affected by the effect of the radium on his throat in 2008, so he can only faintly taste things, and sugary things are supposedly top of the list. Funny that! Sounds slightly suspicious, I know.

The other effect of the radium was that it burnt away nearly all of the saliva glands in his mouth. This left him carrying a bottle of water or a tube of gel lubricant at all times to stay comfortable. He gets distressed if he doesn't have either one of these with him. Naturally. This impacted his time in the oxygen chamber too, as he wasn't able to drink water, coupled with the fact that he's not great with tight spaces. He's done two sessions in the chamber now, but I know he really doesn't like it and we're not sure he'll do it again.

We sit and chat. I start to ask how he is feeling but he says he doesn't want to talk about that. Fair enough. In fact, it's almost like he's read my mind regarding my worries about my work.

'How's the business coming along, hun? You worried about anything from that side?'

I start laughing. He just knows when something needs to be discussed. He's very intuitive.

I tell him it's going great and motoring along nicely but pretty soon we are discussing the very issue that has been on my mind: managing the business with all that is ahead of us.

He gets this like no one else I know. My dad has one of the best, if not *the* best, minds I know, coupled with huge drive and a determination which I admire no end. He is an ideas man and very knowledgeable. His creative thoughts are fantastic. Somewhat unbridled, some might say, but I think it's fantastic and it's just part of his nature.

'This is going to be a tough road ahead of you, hun, but you are well able.'

Ahead of me? Ahead of him, more like. His kindness towards me has me ruined half the time. He's thinking of me when this should all be about him.

'You know that the business has to come first sometimes. You have to keep things running. So don't ever feel you are putting clients ahead of me. I completely understand and *you* need to understand that.'

He continues to tell me how he will be fine and not to worry if I have to take clients over helping him one day. Mum is there. Thank God.

'Don't project too much into the future either,' he tells me. 'It will all work out, and when times get challenging we'll just take them one day at a time, yeah? Don't be worrying now. I promise it will all work out.'

I believe him.

We sit there chatting for nearly two hours before I have to go back to work. He's going to play some guitar down in John's, anyway; they're working on a set-list to play at a gig they have in the Convention Centre. Dad managed to get their band in at some big event there and they are all having a great laugh over this. 'And they're going to pay us!' Dad proclaims proudly. He can't believe his luck! He'll be like a dictator now, I imagine, getting the guys to rehearse till their fingers bleed, till their throats can't sing another note, or they get repetitive strain injury from whatever instrument they are playing. However, that's just who he is!

NOVEMBER 2013

8

STATE YOUR BUSINESS

'Lisa, it's your dad.'

Ha! Still announcing who he is.

'You know, Dad, your name comes up on my phone when you call, and even if it didn't, I know your number by heart so there's no chance in the world I will never not know it's you,' I remind him, *again.*

'I know, I know,' he laughs. 'Habit.'

'So, what's the story?'

'Do you remember the ads we did back in 2011 for the HSE?'

I do, I tell him. Distant thoughts of the HSE's QUIT campaign come forth. Every few years the HSE launches a new anti-smoking initiative and we took part in the last one, in 2011. Three TV ads were made, hammering home the point that one in every two smokers will die of a tobacco-related disease.

The first ad featured a teenager from Kilkenny, Margaret O'Brien, who bravely spoke about losing her mother, Jackie, to cancer when Margaret was just sixteen and her mum was only in her forties. The second ad focused on Pauline Bell, who spoke about her husband, George, who had died from a sudden heart attack at forty-eight. The third ad was based on my father's story. His ad was the 'good news' story of the three: about his throat cancer, how hard the treatment was, how much he could have lost. His message was that he nearly died of throat cancer, but now had a second chance and was grateful to have it.

I hadn't thought about it for ages.

Dad continued: 'Well, funny thing, I was on to a woman called Fidelma Browne from the HSE recently. You might remember her. She was the woman in charge of those ads. She happened to ring when I was leaving St Vincent's a few weeks ago, as RTÉ were looking for someone to do an interview about being affected by a smoking-related disease and she thought I might like to take part.'

I remember Fidelma's name being mentioned from time to time back then, though I'd never met her. I did meet a woman called Steph Green, though only for a few hours in my apartment one evening, when Ciara and I were interviewed and filmed for the ad. She had been the director.

'I told her I've been diagnosed with lung cancer and she couldn't believe it. After the call, though, I had an idea and rang her straight back.'

His voice is so cheerful. I can hear excitement in his voice, which is a breath of fresh air.

'Oh yeah? What was your idea?'

'I just think there's a powerful message in my story. I mean, I haven't smoked in ten years and I'm goi– ... I've got lung cancer from smoking.'

He nearly said, 'I'm going to die.' I know he just nearly said that. Ciara would kick his ass if she heard what he just *nearly* said. But I let it slide. I'm starting to feel it's support he needs right now, not tough love for something he can't do anything about, no matter how much positive mental attitude we all throw at the situation.

I blink, focusing now on what he's actually saying. He thinks there's a powerful message in his story? From the tone of his voice I can tell that, whatever he is thinking about, he has already decided he wants to do it.

'So, there's a meeting in the Glenview tomorrow with Fidelma and her team at 12 p.m. to talk about it. Are you around to come with me?'

I know straight away Mum will not be able for this.

I feel a little caught on the back foot. I don't even have any questions. Everything has been hospital and doctors, and now this is something completely different. A meeting with the HSE? Do they know how sick he is? I don't get it. What could they possibly want him to do in his state?

To be honest, I feel hugely protective of my dad and his health right now, so anyone trying to expend any of his precious energy is an enemy of mine until proven otherwise.

In the end, I cautiously agree. 'I'm not entirely sure about this, Dad, to be honest, but I'll go with you and let's see.'

***

The next day I fly up the motorway in between clients. I'm late. How does this keep happening? I think I'm leaving myself loads of time but before I know it I'm tearing down the road trying to catch up the minutes that have gotten away from me. I throw the car into a space and speed-walk into the hotel. Thankfully it looks like they have just arrived.

Dad walks over and gives me a big hug, thanking me for coming. He wants to introduce me to everyone so I walk over with him to the group of three people standing in the lobby.

'Lisa, this is Fidelma, you may remember her from the last ads. This is Dr Fenton Howell, the HSE's head of tobacco control, and Pearse, who works in the HSE's advertising agency.'

We do the 'nice to meet you's. I can't bring myself to be overly pleasant, which is a bad habit of mine when I'm feeling defensive.

We sit down in old chairs in the front room of the hotel with fantastic views of the valley. Tea arrives. Fidelma, who is clearly in charge, starts explaining the campaigns they run in general, what the various aims are for their campaigns and what they look like when they are finished putting them together. I'm trying to listen but I'm also busy sizing them up. I'm not sure what I'm looking out for exactly but I'll know it when I see it.

'So, that brings us to today, and to how we've tried to respond to Gerry's call and his suggestion about making a new ad about what's happening to him now. Gerry and I have spoken at length about this over the last few weeks, and we have been discussing it with experts here and internationally, and with the advertising agency, to see what is the right thing to do. We have been thinking about whether we should and could make an ad like this, and this is what we have put together so far.'

Fidelma pulls out a large, glossy, A3, bound document. She hands everyone a copy. I open my copy up and glance through all the pages quickly before returning to the first page. I am quite surprised to see images of Dad, Ciara and I – screen grabs from the 2011 TV adverts – displayed on each page, used for the purpose of demonstrating where, in terms of concept, they are hoping to go with this new one. I also notice my long hair. I look so different. Ciara has her fringe. That's long gone, too. Dad looks younger. Healthier. I feel a pang in my heart.

I look back up at everyone as I feel that I am now starting to get up to speed.

Fidelma starts talking. 'Our main concern here is that you are cared for, that you and everyone involved would be okay with what we might do and how we do it. We appreciate it is an unbelievably sensitive time for you all and we are very conscious from an ethical point of view that we approach this carefully. For example, we'd like to check with your oncology team, get their views. But mainly we need to make sure your family would be aware, involved and supported.'

Well, at least we both agree on something, I think, though I don't let my guard down by saying anything aloud. I have no idea if what she just said was bullshit, or if she is being genuine. I am just staring at her at this point. Does she really care about my dad and us and how this is going to affect us? There's silence at the table.

Dad speaks. 'Of course there's huge concern for everyone involved here, guys. Sensitivity must be shown at all times. However, I feel strongly that there is a hard message and lesson in the cards that I've just been dealt – and I think that some people might benefit from hearing about it. I think I could help people quit smoking, and I think this is something we can do together as a family, something I can be really proud of. And now is the time to strike, when I don't look too sick. No one wants to look at a sick man on TV, after all, though the message will still be powerful.'

Because everyone there but me has discussed this at length many times already, Dad included, I feel on the periphery as they continue to talk about this fledgling campaign. I begin to feel uncomfortable; it's hard to hear all this. As they keep talking about what a great opportunity this is to help people, I'm just thinking about what this means for me, for my family and, more importantly, for Dad.

No, I don't like this.

It's at times like this that I wish I were less sensitive. I know it makes me who I am – or so I tell myself – but it can be inconvenient at times like this. I can feel the tears coming as the conversation continues. I'm desperately trying to hold them back. Nope. I can't. There they go, rolling down my face with not a hint of shame off them. *Damn it.* I try to look as stern as possible so they will ignore the tears.

As they continue to talk, I can see that Dad is lit up. He's smiling and looks like himself again. He's so inspiring when he believes in something. It's his voice, though, that shows that he has already committed to this. I can hear the same certainty I heard on the phone. I am both thrilled and saddened by this because I know he is going to jump wholly and soulfully into this campaign and he will want us all by his side. The sadness is there because I fear that he may not get that support. It'll be a tall order for the people close to him, who love him dearly, but who may not want him to exert himself and expend his energy reserves. Some may not want what's to come to be so public, particularly when things are already so tough. Throwing this at them now may not go down well.

I take a breath.

'So what would this mean for us? Who would be filmed, how long would it take?' I dare to ask.

'Well, I'm glad you asked that, Lisa. That's partly what we wanted to talk to you both about today. We've had some ideas, as you can see, about what the ads might sound like, what we would show, who we could talk to. Gerry is adamant he does not want to be shown while very ill, or in hospital, and we agree with that. So, that would mean getting the filming done between now and the end of the year.'

It's November now. *God, filming; this is mad.*

Fidelma explains their general thoughts on what's ahead. The idea they've sketched is to have interviews with Dad and those close to him who are happy to be part of the campaign, as well as following Dad around for a short time, filming him going about his day-to-day life. They would take the same approach as the last time in 2011, recording the footage first like a documentary, and then letting Dad's and our words shape the final content.

She continues slowly: 'We were discussing this earlier this morning. We think it might be about ten days in all, and if we do it, we are hoping to use the same director, Steph Green, and the same crew as last time. At least that way they'll be people that you've all met and, I think, liked. We want to make the duration of filming as short as possible, so it's not too demanding on Gerry and on you.'

Okay, lady. That's the second thing we agree on. A positive for sure.

I have no other questions for now. That really was the only one I felt I needed answered immediately. Others are being answered by the natural flow of the conversation.

I'm exhausted by the time the meeting comes to an end. We say our goodbyes and Dad and I stay back to chat. We go to the bar and have a quick coffee.

'So, what do you think?' His eyes are full of mixed emotions, but I know he's hoping I'm behind him on this one.

I hesitate before responding. 'I don't know, Dad. This could be really tough going. If it's something you really want to do then I'll back you 100 per cent, but let's just think this through some more and chat to everyone about it, okay?'

He nods in agreement.

***

Mum's kitchen table has rarely felt like a battlefield, but today it does. Three very separate battalions: the Yes camp, the No camp and the Indifferents. Each company sits, waiting, watching.

Silence.

The kettle boils. The tension is broken.

'Tea, anyone?' Mum asks.

We all nod.

It seems no one especially wants to make the first move. We've all had conversations with each other about this already, so we pretty much know where everyone stands; we just haven't had an out-in-the-open discussion on it all together.

Dad breaks the silence. 'So, lads. How are we all feeling?'

A reluctance to talk still hangs in the air.

Ciara and I had arrived before Stephen and Dad, and have already chatted with Mum. Ciara is on board with this entirely. She, like myself, feels if anything is going to bring good vibes to Dad's life, then it's a good thing. Even if we all need to hold him up while he's doing it. Dad's big heart and relentless drive means Ciara is rightly anticipating that even when he's too sick to do something he will attempt it anyway and this, she feels, is where we will have to come in.

'Well, I'm behind you in this, Dad. Whatever you want to do, I'm in,' Ciara responds.

Dad nods and smiles. 'Thanks, Babs. I really feel this will be a good thing. It'll bring with it lots of positivity. It'll be good for all of us.'

Now that's where I know Mum totally disagrees. I glance in her direction, where she's still making tea. She doesn't bat an eyelid, nor does she acknowledge that sentence. But I know what she's thinking.

'Steve, how do you feel about it all?' Dad asks.

Stephen is sitting back in his chair. He looks distant and slightly on edge. His life is shooting into adulthood at the moment. I'm constantly in awe of his strides through life. He's

97

had two big milestones happen this year. He got married and his wife is now seven months pregnant. I can only imagine how difficult his heart is finding it to be in two places at once. One life arriving into the family, while another is leaving. He's also started a new role in a big IT company in Sandyford and he's under pressure with the demands of learning a new industry. Besides all that, I can tell he's generally uncomfortable with this conversation. Emotions are not Stephen's favourite indulgence, something that is openly admitted by him and for which he remains unapologetic.

'Yeah, Dad, I'm all for you doing this, but I don't want to be part of it. I'll go to the events or whatever they are but I just don't want to talk or do any interviews.'

Fair enough, I think, though I can't help but feel he should contribute. I had consciously attempted to leave my judgemental side at home, where it can't point fingers at anyone, but it appears it managed to follow me here. I'm conscious I can be judgemental when I feel strongly about something, or if I feel someone is being morally off. As far as I can see, there's a bit of both going on here as Stephen opts to stay neutral.

The teapot is placed on the table and we all help ourselves to the chocolate-chip cookies as Ciara pours.

I reiterate my view on all this. I'm with Dad. I've met the HSE people, and in fairness, although it was almost an out of body experience, I did get a good feeling about them. Dad's vision is so clear and certain to him, it seems wrong not to support it. He's unwavering and adamant that he wants people to learn from his mistake. He's certain we need to try at the very least. But the thing he's unyielding about is the positive energy this will bring us as a family. I'm not so sure about that, if I'm being honest, but I do think it will bring about something good. Somewhere.

Mum finally speaks. 'Well, I'm not sure about any of this.'

Between Dad's chemo and general hospital visits, she is not up for much more. Her stress levels are through the roof and when she gets stressed she gets anxious. Furthermore, although she hasn't said it, she's probably concerned about being dragged into something where she doesn't exactly know her place. They have been separated for two years, after all, and even though they are now acting like best friends, sort of, none of this screams 'normal'. So I get where she's at.

'I know, Delly,' Dad sighs and drops his head. They've obviously had their own conversation about this already.

'Gerry,' she continues, 'I'm just worried about the kids and how dealing with all this' – she points to Dad's humongous pile of medication on the counter – 'in public is going to affect them!'

This is where I get annoyed. We're not kids. We're adults, dealing with an adult situation. Though I suspect I'm probably feeling just as protective of Dad as she is of us. It's a minefield of emotions and layers. But the thought of him going into this arena without us all there to back him up angers me, especially under the circumstances. He'll be vulnerable and subject to the mercy of the press and keyboard warriors. What if someone says something hurtful to him and we are not there by his side? We all need to be on board.

'I'm sorry, Gerry; I just don't like this. I think it's all going to be too much, considering how sick you are,' Mum concludes.

Silence.

'Look, guys. I get it,' Dad says. 'It's scary. It's potentially going to take up a lot of energy and you're worried it'll make me more sick and make a difficult situation even worse by it being so public.'

'Yeah, that probably sums it up,' Stephen agrees.

'But I feel in my soul that this is the right thing to do. It'll bring purpose for me and it might even be a nice legacy to leave behind if it can help even one person,' Dad says gently.

Ciara jumps in. 'Like I said, I am up for this, Dad, but only if you promise to mind yourself throughout. I'm being serious now. If you're not well enough to go to something, then you don't. If you feel you need more help with something, then you say so. Your health *has* to be the *most* important thing, above anything else here.' She's covered a lot of ground with that statement.

'Lisa?' A courtesy ask from Ciara.

'Yeah, Ciara's right. I know you're worried, Mum, but think about the positives that could come from this. Plans will be made that aren't only hospital related. There'll be a bit of buzz about the place. It'll be an opportunity to feel good and to actually do some good.'

'Mmmmmm.'

Well at least it wasn't a complete no.

We continue to thrash out the situation, about the time and energy that we anticipate will be needed for what's ahead, going through every scenario we can think of. The filming, the time it will take, how we'll be affected, how Dad's health may take a hammering, how we all feel about being so exposed after the ads are launched. The scenarios are endless.

A few hours later, after tears have been shed and hugs given, the battlefield is cleared. While a lot of pain undoubtedly sat around that table, it's clear that the room was filled with even more love.

Ciara and I are in full support of whatever Dad wants. Stephen is pretty supportive of it but does not want to be interviewed. Mum, while she is not completely against it, is still heavily concerned that it will do more damage to our family than good.

This, I know, is a hard blow for Dad. Family is important to him and I know he wants all four of us on board. My heart breaks for him, but we will have to get on with it. Perhaps in time things might soften out. At the end of the day you have to respect people's decisions and choices, even if you don't agree with them. Who am I to tell them that they are right or wrong? So I say nothing.

DECEMBER 2013

9

I DON'T KNOW IF I'M CUT OUT FOR THIS

Everything has kicked into gear now that we have given the go-ahead, despite Mum's reservations. The HSE and the production team have been making all the plans and arrangements, including linking with Dad's team at St Vincent's. Dad's phone is ringing constantly. Meetings are being planned. A schedule is being put in place for filming. There's no mention of doing any more chemo right now.

Ciara, Dad and I are going to meet with the crew for a coffee and chat before we start filming. Even though Ciara and I are outwardly encouraging about this, now that it's actually happening I must admit that we are both feeling very apprehensive. The only person who seems completely unwavering about this is Dad.

As Dad, Ciara and I head down to the Italian restaurant in Greystones to meet the film crew, I suddenly notice I'm holding my breath. I'm just realising how important it is that we like these people. What if they are too business-like about this? I hope they know what they're doing.

When we arrive we are immediately greeted by the whole crew.

'Hi guys, so lovely to see you again!' It's Steph. She gives us each a big hug. I hadn't really been able to recall earlier exactly what she looked like, but it's all coming back to me as I hug her back. She's very petite and has a lovely relaxed way about her.

'Hey! Nice hair!' I say, pointing at her hair. It's way shorter now than last time I saw her.

'Thanks! You too!' she responds, nodding to mine.

Steph turns and introduces the rest of the gang to us.

Firstly there's Tamara, the production manager. She has an accent that from a stab in the dark I'd say is Australian, but it could be New Zealand. Steph goes on to explain that Tamara does a lot of the background logistical work and makes sure everything is exactly the way it's needed at any given stage.

Next is Zlata Filipovic, the production assistant. She's much younger than the rest of the crew. She's definitely from Eastern Europe somewhere but I can't tell where exactly. I like her immediately; there's a sincerity to her.

Michael Kelly, the cameraman, is tall with a big moustache and has a slightly hipster vibe going on. What I notice mostly about him is that he seems very relaxed. I could do with a dose of what he has.

Graham, the sound guy, is a good-looking guy. He's a little more reserved than the rest, so I can't make him out fully.

Maybe sound guys are a bit quiet because they have to be for a living? A bit of a wild, on-the-spot generalisation, I know!

Lastly, we're introduced to a guy who looks to be about my age called Lynchy. I'm guessing that's his last name. His role is general logistics guy, which means he'll be on hand to back up everyone. He seems like a lovely chap, too. I notice there's a look in his eyes. A hint of sympathy perhaps?

That's it. They all seem lovely and welcoming, so I decide just to see how this all goes. I'm trying to ease myself into this alien world. The last ads were nothing like this. I literally saw Steph for two hours and that was it. The production around it was nowhere near this scale.

We sit down and Steph talks to us about what the next couple of weeks will look like. Logistically there's a good bit to work out. Very clear communication is required from us in terms of what days we are each free, and at what times, so they can arrange and organise interviewing around our schedules. The plan is for each of us to block off time to be interviewed individually, maybe an hour or so. Then we also have to schedule various times to be filmed together, as part of the background shots to show Dad's day-to-day life – going for dinner, attending a family party, things like that.

This is a bit tricky for me as December is my busiest month of the year and my clients tend to book in at short notice. This can make it difficult to plan ahead. As the meeting goes on and we get further into the nitty-gritty of tying down times, dates and places, I can feel myself getting agitated. I'm hoping Dad or Ciara is getting all this because it's going over my head. Steph is excellent at talking through these things, of course; it's just requiring a lot of thought and I'm currently operating purely on a need-to-know basis. My brain might implode if it's asked to take in information it doesn't need immediately. Just tell me where I need to be and when, and I'll make sure I'm there.

Steph is also expressing how sensitive this all needs to be and that our best interests come before anything else – that we are comfortable with how everything is done is most important. I appreciate that.

***

I'm not in the best of form when I wake up. I hardly slept a wink.

Filming has commenced over the last few days. Dad has been doing his interviews and he's loving the energy and he's loving Steph even more. They have really hit it off. I'm so glad for this because it can't be easy doing those interviews. Feeling connected and safe with the person asking the difficult questions, I'm sure, is paramount.

Yesterday evening, Ciara did her interview. They set up in Dad's apartment and interviewed her when she got back from work in O2 Telecoms, where she deals with inside corporate sales and customer support. It's not her forever job but she's enjoying it for now. I went over to Dad's as the film crew was setting up. I was intrigued watching them transform his sitting room into a TV set. It was not their first rodeo. They had it finished in a couple of hours and were ready to go by 7 p.m., the room transformed with soft lighting, big fluffy mics in the air, light reflectors, the interviewer and the crew. Food was also brought in, which was an added delight. It was dinnertime, so I think most people were pretty ravenous.

Initially, I hadn't been sure whether I should be there for her interview, but Ciara asked me to come for support, so that put my mind at rest. I was in awe of her as I watched her articulate her answers with such thought, while battling through her emotions. If I get through my interview with half as much grace I will be happy. I hope I can speak my truth. I feel so displaced from my normal range of emotions that I'm not sure if I'll be able to talk about anything on a real level. I'm nervous, to be honest, particularly given that the crew are coming over to my apartment today around 4 p.m.

In an effort to get me out of this mood I take out my journal and attempt to write a few things. It helps a bit. Before I close it I notice it's actually been months since I've last written in it, which is very unusual for me, as I've kept a diary for as long as I can remember.

I head off to work and come back. Everyone arrives at the same time. I am having a terrible hair day. It's my turn to have my sitting room turned into a film set. I'm up in my room and the film crew are downstairs doing their thing. I've pre-warned Kat that all this is going on today but I don't think she'll be back anyway. She's with her own dad, who is also not well at the moment.

Oh God, I think, as I try to prepare. There's lots of movement downstairs as they finish preparing the sitting room. I'm starting to panic and feel really vulnerable. My hair is so flat and I cannot find *anything* to wear. My make-up is not great either and I couldn't get my eyeliner the same on both eyes. Plus, I have a cold.

'Lisa, are you doing okay? We're ready whenever you are but there's no rush.' It's Steph and she's standing at the bottom of the stairs calling up to me.

I pop my head over the banisters. She sees that I'm not okay.

'I can only find this bluey/greeney top to wear, Steph. Is it okay?' I hold it up so she can see it. We were told to avoid wearing white, black, stripes or patterns, as they do not appear favourably on screen. But almost my entire wardrobe, I've just realised, is made up of white, black and cream.

'That's perfect, Lisa. You'll look great. I promise it'll look perfect on camera.'

And that's why she's the director. She can see that I'm afraid of all this and, as a result, looking halfway decent for the interview is important to me. Her words provide me with at least some reassurance.

'Let's just ease you into this with a few warm-up questions. Is that okay?'

Okey-dokey. I can do that.

I finish organising myself and head down to the sitting room, where I take my designated seat. The camera is closer than I thought it would be and Steph is behind it instead of in front of it, where, for some reason, I thought she'd be.

You're okay; she's meant to be there. Is my lip-gloss still on? *Yes, you look great.* Are you sure? *Absolutely. You've got this.* Okay.

The basic warm-up questions start. Nothing too major. General information about myself and a few light stories about

Dad's OCD quirks that she'd previously heard about from Ciara. Steph is so professional and friendly. I don't know how she does this job. The interview continues and I talk about getting the news of Dad's cancer and what's been happening since then. I notice the room is getting pretty chilly, though, which is distracting.

Steph gets a little further into her questioning. 'What do you feel is the most important time with your dad now?' I think about this for a minute. I think back on the last few months. It's easy to tell what the important things are. It's all the small daily things, I tell her. Coffees, walks, chats. In my experience, it's not about the big holidays or forced memory making. I get through the question okay but it's hit a nerve.

We stop the filming for a minute. I am starting to visibly shake now – it might be the cold, though I'm wondering if it is actually the adrenaline, but, whatever the reason, it's coming across on camera. Zlata very kindly lends me her grey cardigan. I shake out and rub my arms to warm them up. Lynchy and Tamara leave the room, as it's starting to feel a bit crowded. Tamara says she'll turn on the heating. I'm glad of the interruption. I'm aware that last question exposed a nerve, so I need a minute to mentally cover it back up.

As we restart the interview, I struggle to answer, or even understand, some of Steph's questions. I have to keep asking her to repeat the question. As she probes a little more specifically about my relationship with Dad, I begin to feel alarmed. I'm mentally scouring through my memory banks, grasping for examples or stories of him, or of us together, but I can't seem to recall any of them. Not any good ones, anyway.

The interview is going on and I am talking absolute non-sense now. Ciara's went so well yesterday and now I'm letting them all down with this utter drivel. I'm not even sure what they *need* from me. What makes a 'good' story of him? What story is going to help him make this ad? I have no idea what I'm doing. Am I even meant to be 'doing' anything?

I'm trying to look calmly at the camera but the inner mono-logue going on in my head is loud and is sending me into a complete tailspin. Steph asks me another question. I look at her but I can't answer; the pressure inside me is just too immense.

'I'm so sorry,' I cry. Tears start streaming down my face. 'I feel like I'm talking absolute shite.'

Someone hands me a tissue and I try to catch the tears so as not to ruin my make-up. Steph doesn't falter, although she does look a little confused. Funny. This slight look of confusion helps me. It makes me consider for a second that I might be putting too much pressure on myself here – that maybe I'm not doing as terribly as I thought.

'You're doing great. They're lovely stories you have, Lisa. You briefly mentioned earlier about Gerry escaping from the hospi-tal to go play a gig. Can you tell us more about that?'

I burst out laughing as I blow my nose. He did that. One of the first nights they kept him in St Michael's at the begin-ning of all this, he somehow managed to convince the nurses to let him out. They reluctantly agreed but he had to be back by 12 p.m. so that he could keep his bed. So off he went playing a 'gig' with his hospital wristband on!

Dad, aged twelve.

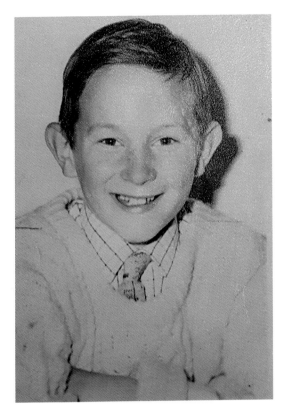

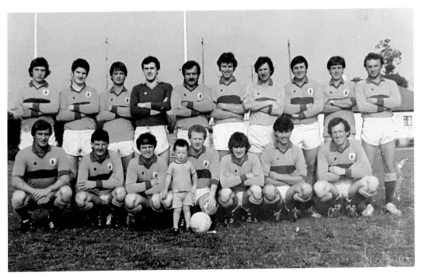

The 1983 Kilmacud Crokes Gaelic football team, with Dad on the far left, crouching.

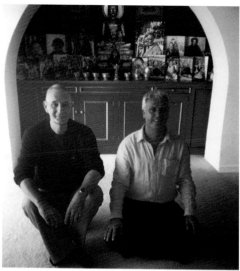

Dad and John in Dzogchen Beara meditation centre in Cork two months before he died.

My husband, Tiernan, and I recreated this picture when we visited a few months after Dad died.

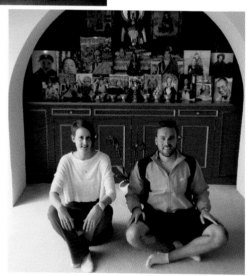

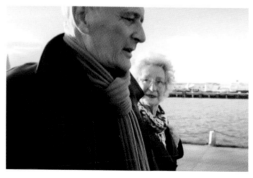

Dad and Nana in 2013.
Courtesy of the HSE

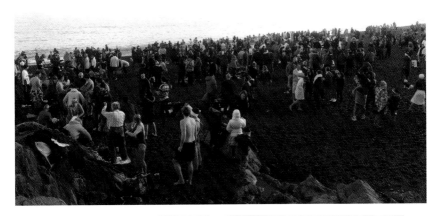

The crowd (*above*) and (*right*) Mum, Stephen, Ciara, me and Dad at Greystones beach on Christmas Day 2013.

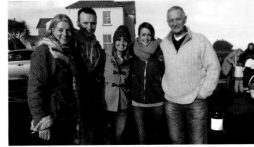

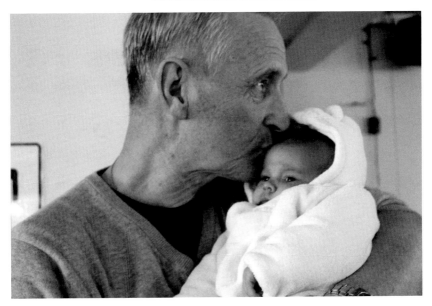

Dad with his first grandchild, Noah.

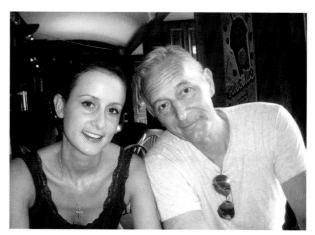

Me and Dad at Stephen's wedding in Guatemala.

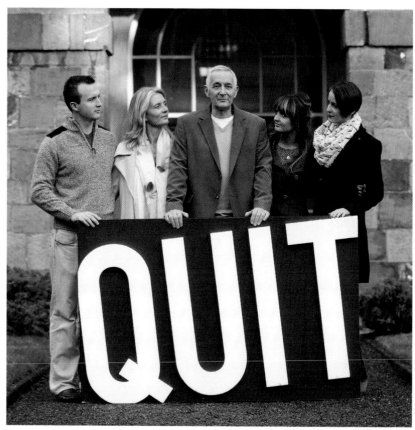

Stephen, Mum, Dad, Ciara and me at the official HSE launch of the Quit campaign ads in December 2013. *Reproduced by kind permission of Robbie Reynolds Photography*

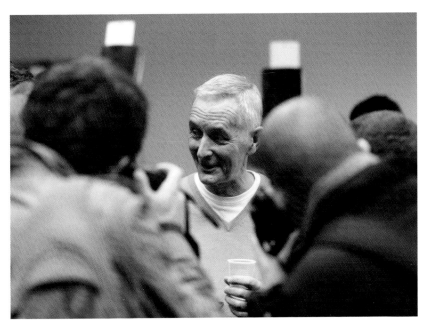

Dad with the press photographers at the official HSE launch of the Quit campaign ads. *Reproduced by kind permission of Robbie Reynolds Photography*

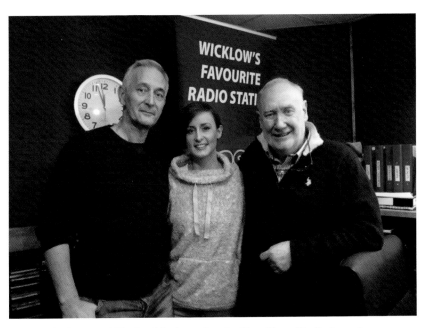

Dad, me and Declan Meehan after the East Coast Radio interview.
Courtesy of East Coast Radio

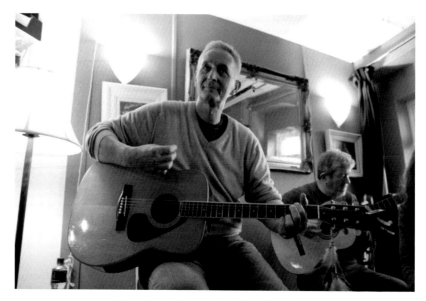

Dad playing his guitar in The Hot Spot.

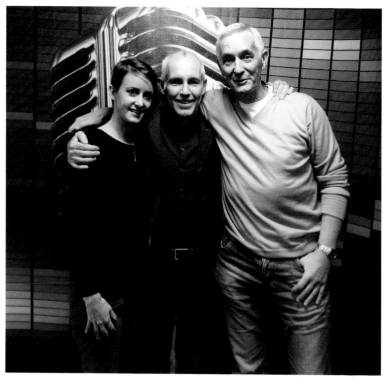

Me, Ray D'Arcy and Dad after Ray had interviewed us for his show.

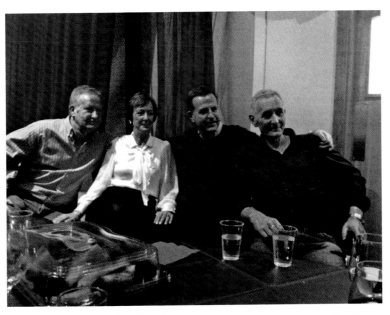

Declan, Rosemary, Paddy and Dad in the green room after *The Brendan O'Connor Show*.

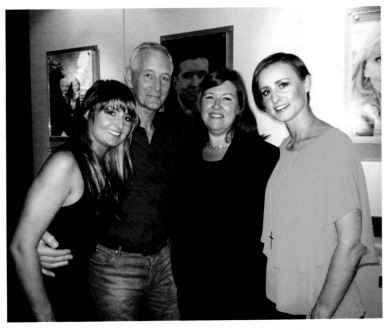

Ciara, Dad, Fidelma and me in the green room after *The Brendan O'Connor Show*.

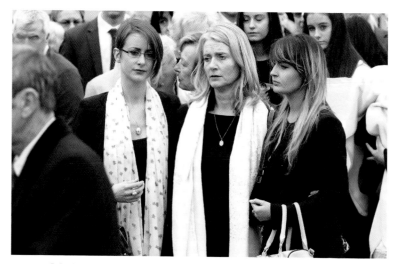

Me, Mum and Ciara at Dad's funeral. © *Collins Photo Agency*

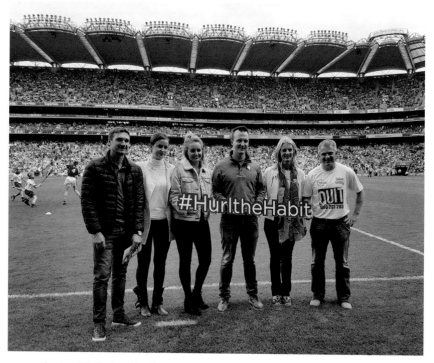

At the All-Ireland hurling semi-final in August 2017, where the HSE's QUIT campaign and the GAA partnered to encourage members to #HurltheHabit. We were invited along and Dad's ads were played on the big screen in front of 83,000 fans. *Courtesy of the HSE*

I start back into the interview but it only continues for another ten minutes or so before we wrap it up. I am too obviously strained and have closed up. I feel terrible, but I'm also glad that they've called it a day.

It turns out it is Zlata's birthday today and she's brought cookies for everyone. Who brings *their own* cookies to *their* birthday? Best person ever.

I have to hand it to the team. I have never seen people work so hard and stay smiling. They have been doing twelve-hour days on this shoot. I know I've had my guard up a lot, but I hope that it's not been too obvious, as inside I am really starting to like these people and feel like they've genuinely got our backs in all of this. Especially after today.

As the crew are clearing up, I change into the fluffiest clothes I have in order to warm up properly. I am relieved it's over. Tomorrow we're due to meet in Bray Bowl to shoot some pool and go bowling. Maybe Stephen has the right idea, I think: to be there for Dad, but just be in the background. I am absolutely exhausted by today and seriously questioning whether I'm cut out for all of this. I really hope these ads are great.

10

ARE YOU HOME YET?

I wake in the middle of the night, drenched in sweat. It's dark and I am too tired to fully address the situation, so I just take everything off and put a towel down. I had a terrible nightmare that Dad had died. That I was trying to talk to him, but it was too late, he was gone. Dreams like this are not uncommon these days.

Thank God he's just in Wexford doing more filming with his old friends from Kilmacud Crokes: Tommy, Gerry and Mick, with whom he played football in his youth. He'll be back the day after tomorrow. I wonder how he's getting on. I hope he's not pushing himself too much, though it would not surprise me if he were.

I had a good chat with him after my spotlight meltdown. He was so supportive. I've been a bit more in the background for the last week or so, but I haven't opted out completely.

Lots more filming has been done. Bray Bowl turned out to be good fun. We've also been to Paddy's house for dinner and the entire Collins family was there, which was really lovely. Dad went for a walk down Dún Laoghaire pier with Nana the other day and they caught some footage of that. They even got some shots of Mum with Dad in St Vincent's a few days ago while she was there with him for his check-up. I think she's secretly happy about that. They also filmed us when Ciara and I met with Dad a few evenings ago in the Italian. They basically just filmed us having dinner and chatting.

Dad was really tired that evening, so we didn't stay long. He's also not eating much, I've noticed. I must make him some smoothies bursting with all things good in them and bring them over to him. Wexford is the last bit of filming. I think everyone is looking forward to relaxing after it all. It's been full-on for all involved.

***

In the morning I get up, have a shower and try to shake off the nightmare. I don't want it following me around all day. I'm also contemplating ringing Greystones Cancer Support. They have been on to Mum about us using their services. They try to help people manage their stress levels during this period. I'm conscious that although there's a tendency to think we can handle anything, in fact we cannot. Me included.

Before all this, I had never actually realised that they offer support to the families/carers of cancer patients; I thought it was just for the patients themselves. Their leaflet, which rests on my bedside table, details a range of support and services from counselling to art therapy classes to all types of massage. I'm already sorted in the counselling department, but I'm heavily considering reflexology. It's done by a local woman called Kim. I've heard that she's great. I feel a bit weird about ringing, though. 'Hi, my dad has lung cancer. Can I have a free massage?'

Oh, just get over it, Lisa, and make the call!

After my shower, I get dressed. It takes a bit longer than normal, as I have to search for clothes that aren't falling off me. Once ready, Kat and I jump into the car and drive down to Kilcoole beach. I find walking in nature or by the sea to be a great way of expending energy. Today there's a lot of nervousness to unload. I can physically feel it in my body. Moving is the only way to calm down. I absolutely love this walk. It's rugged and un-preened and, as you walk along, you have rolling hills and beautiful marshes on one side and on the other you have the sea that displays an unbelievable sunrise on a clear day.

I can usually find some sense of calmness here, but not today. To be honest, I just want this day to be over so tomorrow will come and Dad will be home and I can see him. Have you ever had one of those dreams where a person you love dies and when you wake up you have to ring them or see them ASAP just to know everything is okay? Well, that's exactly how this feels. I just need to give him a hug and I'll be grand. In the back of my mind, though, there's the excruciating thought – that one day in the near future I might have one of these dreams again and he really won't be here. Jesus, I can't bear the thought.

He was meant to go back in for chemo this week but he's decided to take another week off. To be honest, I'm really glad. No part of the process is easy. The build-up to it: all the steroids and tablets he has to take in advance; then the going into hospital, trying to find a vein; sitting there for hours while the poison seeps into his body and destroys everything in its path. There's also the colour change in his skin from the steroids the day or two after the chemo, and the high he is on and, even worse, the subsequent low he crashes to when he's off them. Then there is the violent sickness. The unbelievable heightened sense of smell that can send him into vomiting convulsions. Worst of all, I believe, is the severe constipation. Then there's only the briefest few days of feeling better before the cycle starts all over again. It's so distressing to watch.

I feel bad even saying that it's distressing to watch, but it is. Sometimes I feel guilty about the fact that I find any of this difficult, as it's not me in that chemo chair, but for people who are reading this who are helping their loved one through this process, I think we need to feel that it's okay to find it hard – because it is. Helping someone you love through cancer is bloody hard all round, let me assure you.

***

Finally the next day arrives and I ring him. 'Dad, you home yet?'

'I am, honey, do you want to come over?'

Thank the sweet baby Jesus.

'Yep, I'll be there in two.' Or sooner, if it's physically possible.

All of a sudden it feels like Christmas Day. I don't think I've ever been so excited to see him. This has been building up inside since that nightmare. I cannot wait another nanosecond to see him and get a big bear hug. I throw a jumper on, grab my key and fly down the stairs. I run over to his apartment. I could have driven but I think it's quicker to run, taking into account the unlocking of the car, getting in, driving carefully, etc. I know I am a big ball of emotion here. In fact, I am definitely having a moment. The fact that the day will come that he won't be here for this is hitting me hard. Tears are welling up in my eyes as I'm running across the road. I get to the front door and press the buzzer.

'Come on up.'

I can't utter a word for fear of what would come out. He buzzes me in.

I run up the stairs, taking two steps at a time. I pull open the corridor door and run all the way down to his front door – his is the last apartment. I am aware this all looks very dramatic – not that anyone is even watching except for the critics in my head – but I can't help it. He's left the door open and so I rush in, closing the door behind me. Tears are streaming down my face now. I hear him in the sitting room and go straight in and stop just feet away from where he sits on the couch.

He just looks at the state of me and doesn't say anything. Neither do I. We both know what this is because we just get each other. After a few seconds he stands up and walks over to me and wraps his arms around me. I fall to pieces in his arms. He holds my head to his chest and I sob and allow myself to break down. I feel like my legs are going from underneath me. I can feel by the way his chest is moving that he's crying too. This is possibly the saddest moment I have ever had. I didn't know I had a cry like this in me that was from the depths of somewhere where only pain must reside. I think this is actually the definition of devastation. Yes, that's it. The reality of what is going to happen has hit me like a train and I am absolutely destroyed by it. I am going to lose 'my person' on this planet. My mentor, my friend, my dad and there's nothing I can do about it.

We must be there for five minutes before my sobbing subsides. Snots and tears everywhere.

'Ooops, sorry, Dad.'

I point at his white T-shirt, which now has a big black eyeliner stain. What was I thinking putting make-up on today? I should have known.

'Go away out of that, you're grand. Hang on there.'

He goes and gets me a box of tissues and I gratefully grab a few out of the box.

Holy feckin' moly. I feel like a volcano that's just erupted. I do feel a good bit better, though.

'Sit down there now and I'll make some tea,' he says. 'I have biscuits there as well, but don't tell your mum for the love of God, she'll kill me. The sugar!' he says throwing his eyes to heaven.

I laugh. I won't say a word, I tell him.

He gives me time to blow my nose, gather myself and take a breath. Then he asks: 'Fancy playing some guitar?'

I didn't bring my guitar on my marathon sprint over here, I tell him.

'No problem, you just sit there so and listen to me, myself and I. I know how much you love that.'

We both burst out laughing. He's always playing new songs

he has learned to anyone who will listen. It can get annoying. The funny thing is that he knows this but he doesn't care. He's well able to take the piss out of himself.

'Off you go so. What are you going to play?'

'I've been practising "Walking in Memphis". See what you think.'

For once I sit there happily, even though I'm being forced to listen. Again I remember what Joy had said to me and I get my phone out and start recording. The reason why I am recording this hurts my heart, but the fact of the matter is that I know I will be happy to have this recording in later times. I try and get into the song with him and bring some lightness back into the situation.

As I'm sitting there, watching him, I realise what has just happened here. I grieved with my dad. We both did for both of our losses. For him, it is the imminent loss of his life and his family, as well as his later adult years that he will never get to enjoy. For me, it is the loss of my dad, my person, the loss of the life I would have had with him in it, the loss of him not being there for the big moments in my life, like getting married, having a baby, turning forty/fifty/sixty. They'll be forever bittersweet moments, going forward. This is hard information to take on board, but I feel I am starting to.

I also realise in this moment how brave he is and how selfless it is of him to allow me to do this with him. I think he is, in a strange way, grateful to be there for it too. I think it has given him a sense that he has helped me with these realisations – that I'm not realising them when he is gone. There'll be no man like your dad, for sure, but honestly I feel there is absolutely no man anywhere in the universe like Gerry Collins, my dad.

I start to feel unbelievably grateful for the time we've been blessed to have with him. Blessed to have had him as our dad. No other would ever come close. This thought is interesting because it's new. I no longer feel a strong urge to save him but rather sense that time is of the essence and it is essential we enjoy what time we have left. I feel there's been a shift in my acceptance and I now have a deeper understanding of what is going to happen. I now know on a real level that my dad is going to die. I don't know when, but I know it will be sooner rather than later.

I feel the last of my denial leaving the building as Dad continues to play. I sing louder.

11

THE FIRST AD

We've had huge excitement in the family this past week as we welcomed baby Noah into the world. Karina was in labour for over twenty-four hours, so there was great anticipation as we waited and she gallantly did all the hard work. He is the first grandchild in our family, so no doubt he'll be ruined.

Christmas is approaching. I don't know how to feel about it. Someone said to me in passing recently, 'Make sure you enjoy this one. Christmas is going to be so different for you next year.' That threw me a bit. I hadn't really thought about it like that, though I guess they are probably right. The doctors gave Dad eight to ten months to live, after all. He was diagnosed in June. That only brings him up to next March.

He hasn't done any chemo for the last couple of months and I want to talk to him about this. It's a delicate subject to bring up. He mentions from time to time about going back to do another round in the near future, but the truth is none of us want him to. Having said that, while we don't want him sick from chemo, we also don't want him to die, so it feels like a bit of a lose/lose situation. It's not really our place to say what he should and shouldn't do in this scenario. It's his life and his body. It ultimately has to be his choice. We just don't want him to think that he has to endure more chemo for us.

His general health has been very up and down these days. While it's been great that he hasn't had to deal with the effects of chemo, all the pain medication is starting to take its toll. There are tablets to counteract the effects of other tablets at this stage, and he's taking them all two to three times a day. He's super organised and in an effort to keep track of what he's taking he has put a little system in place for himself: a note pad on which he has drawn columns – one down the left-hand side of the page and one across the top. He has the days of the week listed across the top and the medication listed in the left-hand column and he ticks the boxes when he takes his tablets. It's basic but effective.

One consequence of him taking all these prescription pills is that he's started to suffer terribly with constipation now. They are trying to help him get that under control at the moment. After all, the toxins need to leave the body or he could get very sick. He's also become afraid to eat as a result and that's not good. Something I've noticed about lung cancer is that it seems to suck up any extra energy and picks the weight right off the bones; the person just seems to waste away, so it's crucial that they eat.

At the moment there's a lot to maintain, control, monitor, look out for, try and get into him, or try and get out of him. It goes on and on. In all honesty, everyone is tired at the moment. The filming has taken a lot out of us all in different ways and we're all trying desperately to be there whenever we're needed.

Dad took me aside the other day after I rushed down to The Hot Spot to watch him play guitar, even though I was wrecked after a long week in work.

'Listen, Lisa, you can't be everywhere all the time. You need to realise that, when the day comes for me to go, it'll never have been enough anyway. You can't be running around after me all the time. You need to make peace with yourself in all this.'

This hit me hard, at first, but has helped me greatly. The fear of missing a moment has been a massive weight on my shoulders; after all, the opportunities for regrets are endless. So having Dad's permission to move at a more human pace has helped me manage myself a bit better now and forgive myself for the times I just can't be there.

One event I missed last week was Dad's trip to Mass. Mum had invited him to go to Mass with her in the Carmelite Convent in Delgany. Dad was only too delighted. On the day, however, when Dad arrived to Mum's place, she noticed that he was far from being in his right senses. It was clear he had accidently overdosed on his medication.

Dad was in great form when they arrived at the church. Mum made sure that they sat at the back and she also made Dad sit close beside her, so she could make sure he was okay. After the Mass she wanted to go to confession, whereupon Dad insisted he also wanted to go to confession. Mum told Dad it was best she go in first and he should wait in the pew for a minute. I can see her now, warning the priest in advance of Dad's arrival, worried about what he was liable to say in this state!

Afterwards, Dad talked all the way home about how lovely the priest was. Then, when they reached Mum's and got inside, he fell asleep on the couch. He woke up that evening with no recollection of what had happened.

So it turned into a funny story. We all laughed when Dad retold the story. You just have to laugh; you can't take things like that too seriously, but at the same time we all knew it wasn't really funny. Truth be told, I felt sad. Dad had recently been prescribed Xanax to alleviate physical stress in the body and relieve him of anxiety around his breathing. Although the Pleurodesis had been a success, the tumour unfortunately continues to grow and put pressure on his breathing. This can be very alarming and there's not much more they can do about it. Thankfully there hasn't been another Xanax episode since that day.

In Dad's apartment he has put up a small Christmas tree in the sitting room. He loves Christmas and usually decorates the place to the hilt. This year he's happy with just a small tree for the sentiment. He's also insisting that we do not buy him presents, the underlying message being that he won't be around long enough to get the use out of them. Unfortunately for him we will not tolerate this for a second. His futile efforts to insist that he get no presents are met with 'Shut up, Dad; you are absolutely getting a Christmas present.' The poor man, he's not saying it to be a martyr, but he has to accept that there's no other response we will give.

Today is a bit of a nothing day. I head over to play some guitar with Dad, which I'm hoping he's feeling up to. When I arrive he is really excited. He's just off the phone with Fidelma from the HSE, who has told him that the first ad is nearly ready. They've asked us to go into Windmill Lane Studios in Dublin to view it. They will not put anything on air we are not happy with, so the sooner we see it the better, lest any tweaks need to be made before it's launched.

There are three ads being made in all. The first one will be released the first week in January, aimed at those whose New Year's resolution is to stop smoking. The second and third ones, from my understanding, will be launched around Lent, aimed at those who may try to give up then. We have all agreed that these ads are to be allowed to air for three years. That's fine. If they help, then why would we have any objection?

'So are you free to come in tomorrow, Lisa? Most of the family will be there, and I think they're putting on some nibbles and drinks for us.'

I am instantly hit with a massive smack of guilt. I have a full day of clients tomorrow. How can I ring them all now and reschedule so late? Plus reschedule them to when? I'm fully booked the next day too.

'Crap, Dad, I–'

He stops me in my tracks.

'You're fully booked tomorrow,' he says.

I nod, distraught.

'No problem at all. I don't think Ciara can go either, which I've already told Fidelma. She said she would come out and show Ciara herself, so now you can both do it together.' He sounds completely fine with that, though I can see he's disappointed. So am I. It looks like it'll just have to be that way.

Dad picks up the phone and updates Fidelma. We organise for her to come to my apartment, where Ciara and I will watch it, three days from now.

He hangs up and we continue to chat about tomorrow and what it might be like. Even though all this has taken a lot out of him, in another way it has really created 'good energy', just like he said it would. He's channelling all his thoughts into this, which leaves very little room for the negative stuff. God bless his awareness.

***

Ciara calls over to my apartment about an hour before Fidelma arrives to show us the ad. We have tea and sit in my sitting room. We're both a bit edgy.

The rest of the family and Dad got together with the HSE and the crew at Windmill Lane a couple of days ago and they watched the first ad. It was a big group, including my nana, my aunt and two uncles. Dad's friends who took part in the filming were invited too. It was an emotional evening from what I heard, and I know that Dad talked about wanting the ads to be kept on air as long as possible.

We've heard the ad is brilliant and Dad was very pleased with it, so we know we have nothing to worry about. But I can't help but wonder if, when they say brilliant, do they mean heart-wrenching?

Fidelma arrives with her laptop in her hand. It's freezing out so I have the fire and the heating on in the sitting room. I go to make her tea while she sits down on the couch, chatting to Ciara and setting up the laptop on the coffee table. I finish making the tea and join them.

Fidelma starts by recapping how the other night went. I can tell she is easing us in, which I appreciate – though I'm struggling to listen. I just want to watch the ad. I can feel the tension in both Ciara and I rising, so no doubt Fidelma can too. I haven't spoken to her that much since the first meeting back in the Glenview, but fair play to her for driving all the way out here to show us this. It's 8 p.m. on a Friday evening and I'm sure she could be spending it elsewhere. She does appear to care. She finishes by letting us know it might be hard to watch but it's beautiful.

Then she presses play.

'I wish I was an actor, because if I was an actor, I'd be acting about dying. But I'm not an actor. I am dying. I'm dying from cancer as a result of smoking.'

'I wish I'd stopped smoking sooner. I think my life would have been totally different. I certainly wouldn't be here talking to you today.'

The ad lasts thirty seconds and it's over.

Just like that.

Done.

Silence.

Tears are streaming down my face. Ciara looks pale. I'm not sure where to look. I am just staring at the screen. Fidelma goes to say something – no doubt tactful – but I cut her off.

'Can you play it again?'

She nods and presses play.

Again in thirty seconds it's over.

Silence.

Ciara gets up without saying anything and walks out of the room. I leave her. She needs a minute. I know if she utters a word she will dissolve into tears and she may want to do that in private. It was pretty shocking to watch. I'm so glad we are here and not in Windmill Lane right now.

Tears are still running down my face. Fidelma is right. The ad is beautiful. I know instantly that people will respond positively to it, but it's difficult to look at it from a marketing perspective when it's your father stating he is going to die soon. That he is destined to pay the ultimate price for smoking.

I can see the regret in his face on the screen and it breaks my heart. He knows that he has played the primary role in his own downfall and that he cannot take it back. I feel so strongly for him. It must be very hard to accept a death sentence for the life you lived over ten years ago. I am bursting with admiration for him, as I look at his paused face on the laptop. He is not denying he has had a part to play in his own demise but is now trying to bring some good from the ugly truth. He is trying to save others from making the same fatal mistake. In doing this ad he is showing everyone the bleak and painful truth that awaits most of those who continue to smoke.

'It's brilliant, Fidelma. It's really great,' I whisper.

It's hard to talk right now. In fact, I just want to go to bed.

Fidelma tells me how much time and love have gone into this from behind the scenes and how much everyone in the editing room has fallen in love with Gerry, and us, after watching endless hours of footage. That's nice to hear. I hadn't thought about it like that before.

Ciara comes back in and sits back on the couch. She has very obviously been crying. She hands me a tissue. Fidelma is very tactful and leaves the ad with us for us to watch again when she's gone. She repeats that our being satisfied with how this is working is their main priority. She excuses herself and leaves us to it.

We watch the ad again and cry. My heart breaks for Ciara at this moment as I look at my little sister, who is six years behind me and so has had six years' less time than me with our father.

I hope the ad's really successful because this was really tough for everyone to do. So much hard work has gone into it. It has to be effective. It has to help people. It has to, in order for me to make sense of all this.

***

I head back over to Dad's place the next morning and we talk about the ad. He's in great form. He's really happy with the way they have done it. I tell him how proud we all are of him and we think what he is doing is going to make a real difference.

Throughout this uplifting chat, I still have the chemo on my mind. I feel I have to raise my concerns with him. I don't want to sway his decision either way; in fact, I'm terrified of that. What if I say it and he decides not to do it any more and dies prematurely? I just want to remind him he has freedom of choice. I know I am not the only one who would rather he didn't do any more. It's been so great to see him doing reasonably well again and not be violently ill, bloated and miserable.

'Dad, I want to say something to you about the chemo,' I venture.

'Oh yeah?'

He stops and looks at me, raising both his eyebrows as if to say, 'Go on.'

'Now I don't want you to take this the wrong way, or to let me influence you in any way. I'm just wondering if you've had any thoughts about not doing any more? I'm not saying not to do it, or to do it. I just want to remind you that it's your choice and that there's always room for contemplation with these things.'

There. I've said it. I don't think I offended him.

He looks at me and then looks out the window at the nearby golf course. 'I hear what you're saying, honey, and thank you. But you need to understand that if I choose no more chemo then I am giving up hope and a man without hope is no man at all. I need hope in my life, even if it's just for more time.'

He looks back at me, his eyes reflecting the emotion behind his words.

'Absolutely, Dad, that makes complete sense. Let's knock the next one out of the park when you are feeling up to it so.'

I hope I have concealed my disappointment. His response was not what I wanted to hear, although I understand what he's saying.

'I'm thinking the beginning of January. I want to enjoy the next couple of weeks. The ad is being released on the first of January and there's the launch of it on 30 December in Dublin so I want to be well and able for all that. After that we'll get stuck in and get back into it.'

I nod. At least that's a few weeks away.

'There's also a festival in Glengarriff in June that I really want to play at, so I'm hoping if I'm back at the chemo in January I'll still be doing okay by June.'

That is music to my ears. He loves it down there. The people and the whole traditional music scene light up his soul. The thought of that will definitely help to keep him going.

'Great idea, Dad,' I beam as he picks up the guitar and hits a chord.

12

CHRISTMAS

It's 9 a.m. on Christmas Day and I wake after a good night's sleep to complete silence in my apartment. Usually, at the very least, I can hear traffic outside. This morning I hear absolutely nothing. I lie in bed, staring at the wall for a while.

The silence is a far cry from those households with children this morning, I imagine. I picture the roars and screams of excitement. If they're anything like we were, it'll have been a 5 a.m. start for most of them. I recall our home around this time twenty-odd years ago. How we'd have been sick with anticipation on Christmas Eve, thinking about Santa's arrival. There was no way in hell we were going to make the rookie mistake of falling asleep and missing him. We were determined to meet this man who could make reindeers fly and obviously had more magic in his baby finger than we could ever hope to have in our whole bodies. So, we did our very best to keep each other awake. Come the morning, of course, we'd be literally sick with exhaustion. Sore throats, the works. Our poor parents were completely knackered too – as much from the night of begging, bartering and shouting at us to go to sleep, as well as the fair few Christmas Eve drinks they'd had in our neighbour's.

But this morning I'm snug as a bug and feeling peaceful. I'm consciously starting my day as I mean to go on. No rush. No urgency. Just calm and relaxing vibes as much as possible. Today has the potential to hurt like hell, so I want to avoid any rise in the stress levels and remain in a good space; to be in the moment and enjoy the day.

I sit up and look out the window. It didn't snow. I look at my phone. Not one text. There's a strange feeling in the air. It's not bad, necessarily; it's just there. I throw on some Christmas tunes as I head for the shower. I like listening to music in the shower, as it gets me going for the day. We're having Christmas breakfast in Stephen and Karina's house this morning, but before that we are all meeting down at the Greystones south beach for the annual Christmas Day swim. This is a relatively recent tradition we have incorporated into our family traditions in our adult years.

In my opinion, there is no better way to start this day. It's a magical morning. Hundreds of locals head down between 10 a.m. and noon. There's no exact start time, though. We usually aim for 11 a.m. The energy in the air is always electric, from the people hugging those they may not have seen in a while, to the supporting cheers from friends of those who are braving the freezing cold sea, and of course the screams of those brave people themselves as they run into the icy waters. Some swimmers even dress up for the occasion. Last year, I saw at least three or four Santas, a couple of elves and a rather fabulous-looking Wonder Woman making a break for the sea.

After all these years I still haven't gotten in for the swim, but I am utterly fascinated by those who do. I watch them emerge from the freezing water and while, yes, they look cold, they also look so alive. As if Mother Nature herself has recharged them. It's thrilling. Perhaps one day I'll be brave like them and just go for it. In the meantime I will continue to be a spectator and supply the flasks of tea and hot toddies to brave swimmers. Maybe I'll work up to it next year, I think, by joining the Happy Pear brothers in their sunrise swims in the summer, when it's a bit warmer.

After the visit to the beach, we head up to Stephen's house. Karina's parents are there too and we all sit around their kitchen table and have tea. Noah is the centre of attention, naturally. He's passed around like we're playing Pass the Parcel. He's just so cute everyone wants to have a go. Stephen and Karina are very good at letting us hold him. I imagine it can't be easy as new parents when you watch other people hold your child the 'wrong way', or have the blanket around them incorrectly, etc.

When it's my turn to hold Noah, I sit and look around the table. I feel a mix of emotions as I hold him, particularly when I look at Dad. Here I am holding a baby who is not only new to our family, he's new to the world. He's just about to embark on his life's journey as Dad is coming to the end of his. It's hard to ignore the dichotomy. I'm sure everyone else must be aware of it, too. I'm very grateful to have Noah in my life right now. Even though, as it appears to me, the universe is in the middle of making a swap, I'm glad at least that it's not so cruel as to just take. I love this little boy and it's nice to feel that emotion amongst the uncertainty and pain.

Unfortunately there is just not enough room for everyone around one table for Christmas dinner, so we've split between the two houses. Stephen stays with Karina and her parents, while Ciara, Mum, Dad and I head back to Mum's. We are very much looking forward to the feast that awaits us. Mum's cooking skills are legendary. Ask anyone who's ever been fortunate enough to be fed by her. She cooks everything from scratch, from her sauces to her pastries.

As I watch Mum put the finishing touches to the meal, I think back to the big Christmas dinners she used to cook back in the day with up to fourteen people attending from either the Collins side or the O'Dwyers, or sometimes a combination of the two. The quality and attention to detail she brought to those meals was as on point then as it is now for just us four. She's my kitchen legend.

Mum's place has also been kitted out beautifully for the occasion by Ciara. She has left no spare space undecorated. In the past, she and Dad had a tradition of spending the day together choosing a tree. For Ciara and Dad, the tree had to be perfect. It had to be one where the branches spread evenly outwards from top to bottom and it'd be all the better if it had the Christmassy smell. Both with the same 'tree goal' in mind, they would trek patiently around different places until eventually *the* tree was found and brought home to where I would be waiting, decorations in hand. Even after I had moved out in my early twenties, I made sure to come back for the tree decorating. Some years Ciara's friend Clio would also come up and help. It was a nice ritual.

Today is so different from how it used to be. For so many reasons. But as the four of us sit around the table I realise that different is not always bad. In fact, I haven't felt this happy in a while. I want this day to last forever. We laugh and chat and for the first time in ages forget that there's anything wrong at all. Ciara fills us in on her work, then I fill them in on mine, and Dad fills us in on his band and where they're playing next. Mum is going on about the dinner not being cooked exactly as she'd like it, which is ridiculous, so we respond with lots of compliments and reassure her that it is amazing.

After dinner, relaxing on the couch around 6 p.m., we realise that we haven't exchanged our presents.

'Let's do the presents!' Ciara suggests.

Dad's quickly up off his chair, dying to give his out. He genuinely gets so much pleasure out of giving presents. He just loves it.

We all hand each other our presents and sit down on the couch to open them. I feel quite emotional doing this, which is to be expected, I suppose. There is so much love in this room right now.

There are two presents from Dad for me. We open his presents first so as not to keep him in suspense. Plus he's staring intently at us so there's no choice. I unwrap a small, box-sized gift first. It's a black box and definitely has jewellery of some sort in it. I lift the top of it open and my heart stops for a second. It's a beautiful gold locket with hearts on it. I love it. I hold it up and look at Dad with a big smile on my face.

'Look at the back,' he says, pointing at the locket.

I turn it around and my heart swells.

I'm with you always, Love Dad xxx

I stare at it for a few seconds, taking it in.

I get up off the couch and throw my arms around him.

'Thank you so much, Dad, I beyond love it.'

Words just won't do here. He knows this means more to me than anything. Somewhere in the back of my mind I know this beautiful locket and his words inscribed on it are things that will stay with me longer than he will.

Ciara has been given one, too, I notice. It's a St Christopher medal. St Christopher is known as the patron saint for travellers. As Ciara loves to travel and is often heading off to see various parts of the world, this medal is perfect for her.

I sit back down to open the other present from Dad. It's flat and long and he has without doubt wrapped it himself, given that there's as much Sellotape as there is wrapping paper. I open it and mouth a 'wow'. Well, he has really outdone himself this year. It's a canvas print of the two of us playing the guitar. Amazing. I just stare at it for a minute. What a great moment captured.

Dad still hasn't opened any of his.

'Dad, open yours!' Ciara laughs, pointing to the gifts beside him on the floor.

'Oh yeah.'

He sits down and starts opening them. He opens Mum's first. He's not careful with the wrapping paper, unlike Mum, who could take fifteen minutes to carefully open hers so she can use the paper again.

As he finishes opening it, out of nowhere he bursts into tears and puts his head in his hands. I just stare at him, trying to figure out what happened. He looks up at Mum with watery eyes. 'Thank you,' he says. He stands up and Mum throws her arms around him and she begins to cry, too. 'Thank you,' he says again as he hugs her tighter.

Ciara and I are standing now, staring at the two of them. All this commotion obviously has something to do with the present she got him. I peer around and can see that he's holding a necklace. It's a gold Miraculous Medal. Dad's newfound faith these past months – which up until now I suppose I hadn't thought was that serious – and the fact that Mum herself has given it to him, must be why it means so much to him. No doubt she had it blessed to keep him safe. It is her gift of protection to him. I know he'll wear it every day from here on; it'll be a source of strength for what's ahead.

I start to cry and so does Ciara. We look at each other and we start laughing and crying at the same time. What are we like? Mum and Dad start laughing too and we tell him how fabulous the medal is as Mum puts it around his neck.

I think it's the best present he ever received.

We clean up the wrapping paper mess and sit down to watch a Christmas movie. Dad, of course, falls asleep in about five minutes. Mum falls asleep about a minute after that.

Standard.

Ciara heads out to a party soon after and I head home. Kat is still away with her family. I've been battling a chest infection for the past few days so I'm happy to hit the hay early and let the antibiotics do their thing while I sleep. I'm on my own a lot this Christmas, which on one hand feels strange, but on the other hand, feels very grown-up. Honestly, I'm happy out.

This is possibly the best Christmas Day I've ever had.

13

HERE WE GO

The launch for the first ad is today in the HSE offices at Dr Steevens' Hospital near Heuston train station. It's quite clear as we drive to the launch that Dad is really not feeling well. He appears to be in a lot of pain. I'm in the back of the car with Ciara. Mum is beside Dad, who has insisted on driving. Stephen is driving Karina and Noah in separately.

We're all quiet. It's really unfortunate that Dad is feeling so crap today because I know that he has really been looking forward to the launch. I don't think any of us knows what to expect this afternoon. We're all a bit apprehensive. I'm half expecting a top table with mics so they can ask him questions, but I'm really not sure. They probably told me but I didn't take it in. I doubt Dad has mentioned to them that he's not well either.

As we approach the building, the parking seems a fair bit away. Well, at least for a person who's not at their best today. We look around. There's a man standing near a barrier up ahead.

'Dad, drive up there and tell them you're here for the

THE MAN WHO MOVED THE NATION

conference and you're not well,' I say. There's no point in him
wasting his minimal energy on unnecessary walking.

'Yeah, I'll do that, lads. There looks to be a lot of parking up
past the barriers there that no one is using.'

He drives up and explains what we're here for and the fella
is sound. He lets us straight in so that we can park near the
entrance door.

Dad isn't in great form, for obvious reasons. It can't be easy
to be in good form when you're in pain and also nervous about
speaking publicly concerning your imminent death. We just
help him as much as we can, without helping him too much, as
we know he'll get irritated at being fussed over.

It's a fine line.

The building is huge. We are guided upstairs by staff. The
stairs have beautiful wide steps, which wrap around each side to
the next level. I'm conscious of Dad walking too far, though, so
we take it slowly.

Fidelma is waiting for us at the top of the stairs. 'Hi guys!
Welcome and thanks for coming.' There are hugs all round. She
doesn't look nervous so that's a good sign. Her warm hugs immediately instil confidence. 'Guys, the press conference is happening in this room in here. There's a good few people from
different papers here.'

Although Fidelma doesn't appear to be nervous, I can sense
something else from her that I can't quite put my finger on.
She's definitely choosing her words carefully. I think it's just
because she doesn't want to say the wrong thing. I can't imagine
what it must be like for her right now. She's under massive

pressure today too. She has nurtured this campaign from the very beginning and now it's about to go live. On top of that, she is trying to manage us and our emotional state as carefully as possible. I imagine that's a big ask.

She turns to Dad. 'We'll say a few words, show the ad and they'll probably want to take some photos after.'

Dad nods and smiles.

'Is that okay, guys?' Fidelma asks.

We all nod.

I am starting to feel giddy. I really hope this is going to go okay. She opens the doors to a big room and we walk in.

I immediately see the big screen on a tall TV stand at the top left-hand side of the room. There's no top table, as such; just an HSE-branded lectern beside the screen, which is for the people who are speaking. It certainly looks a little less daunting and formal than I imagined. There are about forty people here.

Fidelma welcomes everybody and gives a speech about the campaign and what it hopes to accomplish. She talks about smoking, how much harm it causes and how, while many people want to quit, it's difficult to get them to take that step. 'We know that ads which are personal and emotional and arresting are the best way to get through to smokers; to help them take that step to quit. That is why we are deeply grateful to Gerry and to his family, who are here today. Their courage and generosity in working on this new campaign is unique and remarkable, and we know that it is going to make a huge difference to the health of the nation.'

She speaks very well. She's calm, cool and collected. I'd love to be able to speak so confidently like that some day, but public speaking is not my forte. When she finishes she introduces Dad and us. People look over, some nod. I'm not entirely sure if we're meant to do anything so I half smile and nod back. Thank God we don't have to say anything.

Then they dim the lights and show the ad.

We, as a family, stand close together for this. It's so strange to see ourselves up on a big screen. It's like people are watching us through our living-room window or something. It's all a bit surreal.

The ad finishes and there's a big round of applause from everyone in the room. I look around and people are smiling and clapping hard. It appears to have been received really positively. There is definitely a lot of emotion in the room.

After the viewing, there are some other speakers from the HSE and then Dad is invited to say a few words. He is proud, he tells the audience.

'There were three reasons I decided I wanted to do this – firstly it was for myself, a positive thing for me to invest my energy in while dealing with my cancer. Secondly, I thought it would be good for my family, creating something powerful and meaningful for my kids to look back on. And finally, there's the point that if even one person stops smoking because of what we've done, then it will all be worth it for me.'

After the formalities, the press instantly swarms around Dad. Cameras flash and questions are asked. I see him come to life in the limelight. He's no longer holding his ribs. He is soaking up the positive energy. I can see it in his animated eyes.

I have to hand it to him – he's a natural. You can't help but love him. He's the most relatable person I know. As I see him answering all the questions, I beam with pride. It's such a brave thing, to talk so openly about his situation. It takes guts. It also lets other people speak freely to him about it, which is fantastic for everyone.

The interviews finish up and Fidelma takes over again. 'Right, if you could all follow me downstairs we can take some photos,' she says, guiding people outside to the courtyard.

A big QUIT sign appears from somewhere and we are asked to stand behind it. As the photos are being taken, I'm really not sure what to do. Should I smile? Would that be weird given the reason why the photos are being taken? No, don't smile. I'll try a straight, friendly face, *whatever that is*.

I sigh with relief when we take a break, though Dad is quickly whisked away for more photos and interviews.

Fidelma appears beside us. 'Lisa, Ciara, *TV3 News* are here and they'd like a word with you. How would you feel about that? Your dad has just done an interview with them.'

Oh God.

I did not expect this. I didn't even realise Dad had done an interview with them. There's so much activity buzzing around us. I glance across at Ciara and she looks how I feel – a bit unsure, to say the least. The news? How many people will watch that? What do we have to say that people want to hear? This is all mental, and a tad terrifying. I really have no idea what to say. But if it helps to get Dad's message out there then I suppose I should try. Hopefully they'll just ask straightforward questions.

Ciara and I agree to do the interview. Suddenly there's a big sponge microphone in front of us.

We speak and it's done before we know it. It lasted two minutes max. It wasn't so bad. My heart was in my mouth for most of it and God only knows what either of us said, but hopefully it was okay. I'm glad that we did it, and that we did it together.

I look over and see Mum with her arm around Dad. He looks unwell again. I look at her and she gives me the nod that we're going. We thank everybody and leave. Mum walks ahead to the car, gets in and drives it over to where the rest of us are waiting at the front entrance, so Dad doesn't have to walk. In the car we can see that Dad is in a lot of pain. More than usual. Mum drops Ciara and me off home and brings Dad to the doctor.

Morphine painkillers are not something given out lightly, so when I hear that's what he has been prescribed by the doctor I can't help but cry. Poor Dad. I hope he doesn't need them often.

JANUARY 2014

14

WE'VE WON

In one week it feels like everything has changed for the better. There's a strange triumphant atmosphere surrounding us. It feels like Dad has somehow managed to beat cancer, like he has seized his life back. He's no longer feeling sick and having all his time consumed with hospital appointments. He has squashed all that by giving new meaning to his life. Filling it to the brim with a higher purpose with this campaign. He did it. He has won. We are in awe of him.

Dad rings me. 'Lisa, you're not going to believe this.' It's clear from his tone that he's finding something amusing. 'Fidelma just called and East Coast Radio, Today FM, Newstalk and even a few others want to do an interview with us!'

He laughs down the phone and I laugh with him.

'Well, well, you're quite the star these days, Dad. Don't forget us now when you're in Hollywood rubbing shoulders with all the A-listers!'

'I'll try not to, honey, but you know yourself: when you've got it, you've got it!'

The ad has been released across all forms of media for a full week now: the radio, the newspapers, all social media platforms, online news pages like *The Journal* and, of course, it's on TV. Kat and I have a huge flat-screen in our apartment but the irony of it is we rarely ever turn it on, so I haven't actually seen it on the TV yet. I understand it is on every hour, though.

Never did we imagine that the ad would receive this type of response. It's been absolutely insane. My inbox is full of kind and loving messages from people. I haven't had a chance to reply to half of them yet. The empathy from other people is incredible. The fact that people, especially people who don't know us, have taken time out of their day to send a message just blows me away.

'Listen, I think you should come to East Coast FM tomorrow and do this interview with me,' Dad says. 'I think it will be really good for you.'

Ah now. Where's he going with this? Public speaking is really not my bag. I'm a much better cheerleader.

'Dad. I really don't think so. I mean, I will certainly come with you and support you all the way, but this is your gig. I don't think I can do it, I'm sorry.'

I imagine the questioning. I wouldn't have a clue what to say.

'So Lisa, your person in this world is about to die. How do you feel about that?'

'Ah, you know, it's not ideal.'

'I know you'll be nervous, hun, but I really feel you need to do this. All this is going to land on your doorstep when I am gone and I want to prepare you.'

All this? I suppose the response to this ad compared to the

one in 2011 is massive, though I'm still not exactly sure what he means by 'all this'.

'Please don't say *gone*, Dad!'

I guess he hasn't completely forgotten he has cancer.

'I'm sorry but I feel this is very important for you. I will be right beside you and we can do it together. If you get stuck just look at me and I'll jump in and you can do the same for me. We'll be like a tag team.'

Silence. I'm thinking.

'Okay, Lisa, look you don't have to, just have a think about it overnight. I'll be leaving at 9.20 in the morning and I'll ring you before I leave and see how you're feeling then, okay?'

'Okay, Dad, I really don't think so but I'll talk to you then. I'm really happy, though, that it's gotten such a great response. You did an amazing job.'

And I am so happy for him. It wasn't easy to do. So much effort from everyone went into this ad, so I'm pleased that it's gotten such a positive response.

***

The next morning I am up, showered, dressed and ready to go. I've decided that I can't have him doing this on his own. I am in jeans and a snug, fluffy top Ciara got me for Christmas. If I am going to do this I am doing it as me and in clothes in which I am comfortable.

My phone rings. It's Dad. 'Well?' he asks.

'Collect me. I am ready to roll,' I say as I throw on a bit of clear lip-gloss.

'Great stuff altogether, see you in thirty seconds.'

I can hear in his voice that he's chuffed. He's outside in less than thirty. I jump in his car. He greets me with a big smile and a hug. I'm so nervous, I can't quite muster up a matching smile just yet. I think I'll reserve that for after the interview, so long as I don't spontaneously combust on air.

Dad does most of the talking on the way in. I stay quiet so I can keep myself calm. When we arrive into the East Coast Radio studio, which is only ten minutes from us, the receptionist is very friendly. While we are sitting in the reception area, waiting, Dad needs to refill his water bottle, so he pops off to find some water. While he's away, I try to relax a bit and loosen up.

A few minutes later they bring us in to meet Declan Meehan, the DJ who will be interviewing us, during an ad break in the show. He invites us to sit down and then, after playing Dad's ad, he introduces us on air.

I am terribly nervous and I can tell Dad is a bit now too. Declan starts by asking him about the campaign and, like a pro, Dad starts telling him how it came to be. He's so good with words. My breathing starts to return to normal; it's relaxing just listening to him speak.

They continue to talk about Dad's smoking history, how he started because he thought it was cool and how there was a lack of awareness in his younger days regarding the negative effects of smoking. They then speak about how Dad made the decision to stop smoking ten years ago. Dad's now telling him how he found out he has terminal lung cancer. He explains how most of the time he – and the rest of our family – choose to be in denial about the fact that he's dying. If he went around every day thinking that he's dying he wouldn't get out of bed, so, instead, we all choose to believe in hope and we are grateful that we have time to create new memories together in whatever time he has left.

Declan asks me how I feel about this and if Dad having cancer has changed my life in terms of trying to hurry big life events like getting married, or bringing forward any other big events so Dad can be there for them. I like this question. I laugh and answer that we did actually take a holiday to try and make our time together more special. But the pressure to create amazing memories that you're meant to have forever after he's gone was ridiculous. We all ended up killing one another and not talking for most of the week! So we realised then that forcing that kind of thing just doesn't work. For us anyway! So, instead, we just enjoy the small things together and, as cheesy as that sounds, it's the genuine, honest-to-God truth.

Declan asks me whether I think it might be easier to have Dad die suddenly from a heart attack so I don't have to watch him die slowly from cancer. I laugh at this question. It must just be human nature to wonder this because he's not the first one to ask me that question and I've asked myself the same thing many times too.

I tell him that I would choose the long goodbye. Maybe it's selfish of me, but I'd rather have the time to say the things I want to say and time for him to do and say the things he wants to do and say. It gives everyone more time to get their heads around it (if that's even possible) and gives people time to have those moments with him that they may not have had before. We always think there's more time, so when you know you've got a deadline it prompts you to say what you may have always thought but have never actually said aloud.

We laugh about how I find myself filming him chopping vegetables and doing other random things, and getting him to play the guitar. We laugh about how we still argue about things, and how we argued only yesterday, but we make up quickly and try not to let things drag on. It's not easy, when emotions are running high, to keep things on an even keel all the time. Understanding and empathy are called on a lot.

Dad finishes the interview by reinforcing his message that he doesn't see any positives in smoking. He urges people who are not smoking not to start. For those who have already started, he tells them to stop. Declan thanks us both for coming in and plays the ad once again to close the interview.

As the ad is playing, the mics are muted and we stand up to say goodbye, thank Declan and shake hands. The receptionist comes in and asks if they can get a photo of us with Declan so they can put it up on their Facebook page along with the interview.

We get out of the interview and crack up. It felt great to be in there with Dad. We're on such a buzz! Plus the interview went really well, which just adds to the excitement. It went on for twenty minutes, though it felt like seconds. We laugh and chat about it the whole way home.

What a day! I'm so happy. More good energy!

15

FAMOUS

More requests for interviews have come in from newspapers and TV shows since the East Coast interview. *The Brendan O'Connor Show* and *The Late Late Show* have both invited Dad on their TV shows. We've gone onto *The Ray D'Arcy Show* on Today FM and I've done a national interview with him. It went very well, I must say – I actually appear to be getting the hang of this.

Ray and Dad knew some of the same people, which was a nice icebreaker. The response from the public to that interview was great, with some people texting and emailing fantastic feedback and positivity. Dad has gone on Newstalk too, which was another great success. The papers have printed a lot about the campaign and done interviews with Dad. I did one interview by myself the other day and it came out as a two-page spread. It's just the craziest thing to see us all in the papers.

This brings me to this evening, where we are due to be picked up by a bus any minute now. Dad is being interviewed on *The Brendan O'Connor Show* and RTÉ have organised the bus to collect us all.

Mum is more than delighted – not because he's going on TV, but because he's finally decided what to bloody wear. She spent all week in and out of the shops with him, helping him find the right thing. He's so fussy about his clothes. He knows what he likes and will not deviate from that.

A few of my girls have come with me, as have Ciara's. I am so appreciative of their support. They have been so amazing and by my side through all of this. I get great strength from their love and positivity. Stephen, Karina and Noah are all here too, suited and booted, ready for the show.

The only downer today is that, unfortunately, Dad really is not well. He doesn't want to take many painkillers in case they make him dopey and we have a 'church episode' again. He wants to speak as clearly as he can so he can get his message across. He's just really nervous. Everyone is feeling it.

'I just hope I don't fall when I walk on. Once I get to my seat I'll be fine,' he says at one point.

There's no particular reason for him to fall, although he does have a natural tendency towards clumsiness, which has given us all many reasons to laugh in the past. To be fair, falling is not usually one of the problems; it's more likely to be dropping and breaking things, or standing on things.

We arrive into RTÉ and are shown to the 'green room'. *Guess what!* This room is not green. In fact, it's burgundy, with nice lighting. *Who knew!* There are drinks and nibbles for everyone. *Don't mind if I do!* Other guests from tonight's show are here already with their friends and family. Paddy, Dec and Rosemary arrive not long after we do. Team Collins are out in force.

Brendan, the man himself, walks in and says hi to everyone and briefly goes through what they might talk about during their interviews. Dad is chatting away to him. We're all standing near; I can hear Dad having a laugh with Brendan, which puts me a bit at ease. At least he won't be walking out onto a stage on national TV to talk to a man he can't chat easily to.

It's at this point that Ciara also heads off to get mic'd up. During the week a researcher of the show rang and asked would one of the family members answer a question. Ciara felt that this was something she'd like to do. Everyone was so proud of her, Dad in particular. It's also nice for them to do this together and I'm also delighted it's not me. Radio is enough for me, thank you very much.

Soon after, we're asked to take our seats. *Here we go!* We wish Dad the best of luck and we head out, leaving him in the green room to wait for his interview slot. Mum, Ciara and I are seated in the front row of the audience. The rest of the family are in the row behind us and the girls are placed in rows further back. Ahead of us is the stage and on it is a long purple velvet couch, which curves slightly to ensure Brendan can see all his interviewees should the couch be full. Brendan is sitting behind his desk facing the couch and has cue cards in his hands. I assume they have all his questions for his guests this evening and are in order of guest. *Do not shuffle.*

I can't imagine it's an easy task – to interview people. People are all so different and each of Brendan's guests is on this show for different reasons. Take Dad, for example. Normal guy meets abnormal situation equals public speaking on national TV.

I think there'd be a lot of people who would end up sitting on that couch and freezing. It's not like they are famous people used to talking in front of crowds. Some might be but not all. So I reckon, for that reason, to be a good interviewer you have to frame the questions in the right way and maybe even carry the conversation should someone freeze. If it was me, I reckon I'd take flight. *Gone. See you later. I'm outta here. Send me on the minutes.*

The show starts with an introductory act, which is some guy telling jokes. I am not taking it in. Flashes of Dad falling keep flicking through my mind. *Go away!* What if Dad does fall? Should Mum run up and pick him up? He's not light! No. It'll have to be Brendan; he's the only one big enough and he'll be closest. What if Brendan isn't nice to him and asks him difficult questions? *I might actually throw something at him.* What if this doesn't go well for him? He's really not well and is in a lot of pain tonight; what if he's just not able for this? *Oh shit, mayday, mayday. Panic stations!*

'Lisa, are you okay?' Mum puts her hand on mine. I think my eyes must be bulging out of my head. Ciara is sitting to the other side of me and all I can think is thank the sweet baby Lord Jesus she is answering that question tonight. I might de-liver vomit instead of words if I had to talk.

I turn to Mum, grit my teeth and do a weird fake smile.

'He. Is. Going. To. Be. Fine,' Mum says. Her very clear, defi-nite and reassuring words help. She keeps her hand on mine as she looks back towards the stage. I know there are cameras filming but I'm really hoping they're not on us right now. I'd say I look demented.

Brendan is now ready for Dad and starts to introduce him. My heart is literally in my mouth. In fact, if I reach into my mouth right now I bet you my heart would be there. I cannot remember a time that I felt *this* nervous. I see Dad begin to walk out. *Shit. Right. This is it.* The audience claps. Dad's smiling as he walks and Brendan gets up to shake his hand. *He's okay. He's okay.* He sits. *Thank you God, he's okay.*

Brendan continues to talk and welcomes Dad as a former Dublin footballer. Dad laughs at this introduction. He lined out for Dublin in 1980 but he was on the bench. He's been a Kilmacud Crokes man all his life. Dad has GAA in his blood. His own father was a well-respected man within the community and a founding member of Kilmacud Crokes. Dad started playing as soon as he was old enough and his father was present at every match. Funnily enough, Dad always said he was a better hurler than he was a footballer, but after suffering a serious injury when he was nineteen, he lost his nerve for hurling and concentrated all his energy on football. He also played for Oatlands College in Stillorgan. In recent years Oatlands reached their centenary year. As part of their celebrations they chose a team made up of the best fifteen players who had passed through the school over the last one hundred years. Dad was chosen as one of those fifteen players and was placed in the midfield position. He felt honoured.

'So, Gerry, how are you doing?' Brendan starts.

'Well, Brendan, as you know, I'm dying from cancer. But, to be honest with you, hearing you call my name there when I was backstage, I think I almost died of a heart attack on the spot!'

Everyone laughs. 'But other than that I'm doing okay, thanks.'

His joke eases the tension in the air.

'And do you know how long you have left to live, Gerry?'

Dad explains how he's been given eight to ten months to live, but since he's fitter than the average male of his age, he's hoping he'll get a bit longer.

'Do you yourself realise you're dying, Gerry? If you don't mind me asking.'

Dad shakes his head. 'No, Brendan. As far as I'm concerned, I'm not dying. I'm in denial for the most part. If I were to fully think that I am dying, I don't think I could get up in the morning. Having said that, I'm in pain where the tumour is, so I know it's there. I'm also sick from the treatment, so I know I'm having chemo for cancer, but still I don't allow them in mentally.'

Brendan changes direction now, taking Dad back in time as he asks how he got here.

'I started smoking when I was seventeen. It was cool back then. Even in the top programme of the day, *Happy Days*, the Fonz had cigarettes in his sleeve pocket to make him look cool. All the smoking campaigns back then were pro-cigarettes, not anti-them. That's just the way it was back then.'

I can't imagine living in a world where there are campaigns that actually promote smoking as a good thing for you to do. But then again, we do currently live in a world where alcohol is still widely promoted. In time, will we look back on this period with the same appalled reaction?

Dad talks about how he started smoking a few cigarettes here and there when he was seventeen and over the years this gradually increased until he was smoking the shameful number of sixty cigarettes a day by the time he was thirty.

'But then, Gerry, you gave them up. When was that?'

'Yes I did, Brendan. It was a big ask, as I was completely addicted to them. But it's been ten years now since I've smoked a cigarette, so it was a shock to get the news that I had lung cancer, and that it was terminal.'

He continues to talk about how he managed to eventually give up smoking in his early forties. How, in the end, he just went cold turkey. After he stopped smoking, he quickly noticed that his body, now free from nicotine, began to demand a healthier lifestyle. This is when he decided not to drink any more. And then he started to join Mum with her hill walking. They would go off for days to various parts of Ireland and trek up a mountain. He particularly loved heading to Glendalough in Wicklow. Even on a windy, rainy day he would put his wet gear on; he just loved being out in the elements. He never would have done this if he were still smoking, he admits. Smoking kept him in a perpetually unhealthy lifestyle. He explains how, from the hill walking, he then got into boxing with Stephen. He also loved that and has been doing it ever since. The boxing was heavy going physically, and it was then that his body really started insisting that he address his diet. He bought cookbooks and learned about nutrition and about how to better fuel his body for the training he was doing. He was in his new and improved element. 'Sure I'm nearly a monk now, Brendan!' he laughs.

Next he talks about the treatment he's been having and the medication he is on and the effects of that on the body. 'I'm doing maintenance chemo now, and I'm on two morphine tablets a day for pain from the tumour. Initially I was on chemo once a week every three weeks, but we've expanded that to every four weeks now, as I wasn't getting enough "well" time during the recovery,' he says, referring to the time where he is well enough to go out.

Dad continues, 'Not to mention the anti-sickness tablets can give you terrible constipation, Brendan. It's no joke. Anyone who's gone through chemo will tell you that.' He laughs, shrugging his shoulders.

Ciara leans towards me and whispers through the crack of her mouth, still smiling and trying not to look like she's talking, 'Did Dad just mention constipation on national TV?'

'Yep,' I reply in the same fashion, still staring straight ahead.

'Fuck sake,' Ciara says and we both try not to burst out laughing.

That's Dad. He just tells it as it is. In that moment – even as I try to stifle my laughter – I am full of admiration for him. He speaks so openly about what many of us pretend never happens.

Brendan then leans forward slightly and shuffles his cards. 'Gerry, do you mind me asking, do you blame yourself at all in all this?'

Dad doesn't even blink. 'I do, Brendan. Absolutely. If I could take back all those cigarettes I smoked I would do it in a heartbeat. It's terrible and I have to live with that.'

I'm in awe as I watch him up there, wearing his heart on his sleeve; it all starts to make some sort of sense. Over the years I know Dad has searched to find himself at different times. I think many of us who think deeply do. Big burning life questions, such as who am I in my entirety? What is the point of our lives here in this world? Am I living my life as I should, as I was born to? What is my purpose here?

As I stare at Dad, I think perhaps he is fulfilling his purpose now. Not to take away from the life he has lived up to this point, but I feel a sense of destiny being fulfilled right now, both in this very moment and during these past few months. As I listen to him speak, it's like the words he naturally chooses are meant to be said. Like a script from an inner source. His soul, perhaps. He is without doubt on a profound and purposeful journey, one we are all watching.

As the interview comes to a close, Dad asks to say a few words. 'I want to thank my family and friends from the bottom of my heart for all their support and love. There was a two-week filming period there that was tough going on them and I under-estimated the level of distress it would cause. They were amazing and I want to thank them from the bottom of my heart.'

It blows me away that he can think of us while he's up there, talking on national TV.

He stops for a second and looks directly at Mum. 'I also want to thank Delly. You see, Brendan, when you're sick you're the star; even if you're vomiting on the floor, it's all about you. But someone has to clean that up, someone has to listen to you, manage you physically, emotionally and mentally. And Delly has done that for me. So I just want to say I love her loads and thank you.'

A big round of applause bursts out from the audience as a tear rolls down Mum's cheek.

Brendan has one last question, for Ciara. 'This must be an incredibly tough time, but you must feel very proud of your old man?'

I hold my breath.

'Yeah, absolutely. It was probably a bit tougher than any of us expected when we started out in all this, but to say we're proud doesn't even cover it. The whole point of this is to encourage people to stop smoking, so if even one person quits then it'll have been worth it.'

Another big round of applause. So graceful and brave; I'm so proud of her.

The show ends and we all head back into the green room to see Dad. He's on top of the world – as he should be. He has done himself and everyone else so proud. I am beyond thrilled for him.

'Daaad! You said constipation on national TV!' Ciara and I are slagging him.

'Yeah, so what? Tell me one person who has never been constipated!'

Touché!

We all stay in the green room for a while, drinking and chatting about the interview. We're all giddy and delighted with the buzz. The energy is electric. John, the girls, Ciara and I decide to go back and see if we can stand on the stage, for the craic. The best reason to do anything! There's no one about so we go for it and start pretending John is interviewing us. Prime photo op. We all take turns to be the interviewer. There's a few props around which we also take full advantage of for some more photos. *I hope no one sees us!*

After an hour or so the evening winds down. It's getting late and Dad is in pain. He's also taken a few painkillers now that the interview is over, so he's starting to feel a bit drowsy. He needs to get to bed. He'll be wrecked for a few days after this.

He was supposed to start doing chemo again last week but he couldn't do it because he would have been too ill to go on TV. He's due to start next week instead. But that's a worry for tomorrow. Now we just need to get him home and hopefully he'll sleep well.

FEBRUARY 2014

FEBRUARY 2011

16

RESPITE

'I've ordered a beautiful bunch of roses for your mum!' Dad announces, delighted with his Valentine's Day effort. Not only has he managed to order them on time but he wrote a lovely message too, apparently. Mum will be chuffed. She loves roses because they remind her of her own mum, who used to have lots of rose bushes that she cared for in the garden.

It's been a rough couple of weeks. Dad went back to hospital and started chemo again. He just did one session but it has hit his body hard. His whole system has seized up. He is very bloated and uncomfortable. He is afraid to eat because he cannot go to the loo and empty his bowels. This is obviously not good because he needs to eat to keep up his strength and keep the weight on him.

The tension of what's happening at the moment is getting the better of everyone. The fact that he's in so much pain can make him snap and sometimes I find myself snapping back. I'd love to say I'm able to contain myself but that's not always the case. The fact that we fought over something ridiculous the other day makes me feel even worse. We made up that night via text and followed up in person the next day with a hug, but I regret it happening in the first place. I should be more under-standing. The man is not well.

We're all just trying to do our best but I still feel bad. In fact, I'm not sure I can feel any worse right now. It seems end-less sometimes – this constant feeling of guilt that I'm carry-ing around with me. I especially feel guilty if I'm in any way having fun. That means any sense of excitement equals copious amounts of guilt and self-flagellation. I feel guilt if I'm not with him. I feel guilt if I'm with him and he's too sick to talk because I think he wants me to go. Sometimes I get bored hanging around his apartment and leave, which brings about more guilt that I didn't stay with him. Basically I'm on a steady diet of guilt for breakfast, lunch and dinner. Brought to me by me. I can't let myself get excited about anything in life right now. Absolutely not. Until Dad is feeling better life must remain beige. Full stop.

Palliative care nurses came to his apartment last week and are now on hand to help him. At first I was shocked to hear that they were here. I thought they were just for dying people. The last time I heard of palliative care nurses was around the time my grandad – my mum's dad – was dying at home. But Mum insists that they're just here for Dad's pain management. Thank God.

I met one of them for a few minutes the other day. She seems grand, but I don't really want to get to know her. I'm hoping she won't be needed much longer. He'll be getting over this chemo session soon, so once he pulls up out of this they should no longer be needed. That's it, though. After this, no more chemo. I don't care what he says. This is no quality of life for any person. It's barely a life at all. He's in bits. I don't care if he's a man without hope, at least he'll be a man without severe constipation!

Right now they are trying to help him get that under control and get things moving for him again, but it doesn't seem to be working very well, or maybe it's just not that simple. They're getting him to take different tablets and use suppositories at night. These are pretty hard core and should be blasting anything out of the way, but they don't seem to be working. It breaks our hearts that he's here on his own at night when he's going through all this. I wake up during the night sometimes and stare at my phone. Just in case something happens and he needs me. Sometimes I text him. Sometimes he texts back. Sometimes he doesn't. I hope he's asleep when he doesn't and not in a bad way lying on the bathroom floor.

I ring him in the morning to see if he's okay.

'I'll bring you over a smoothie, Dad. I made it this morning.' Hopefully he can sip away on that and it'll get some nutrition into him.

'Great, thanks, could you pick me up the paper on your way over?' He hasn't been able to go out the last few days. 'Also, Fidelma rang and they have the second and third ads finished and ready for us to watch. They're going to come over tomorrow evening to show them to us. Are you around?'

I am and it seems Mum, Stephen, Ciara, John, Rosemary and Paddy are too. Rosemary came up from Limerick this morning and she'll be staying with Dad for the next week. I am so relieved she's here. Just knowing that she will be with him 24/7 is very comforting. They have a special bond as brother and sister. They're very alike. I know they will both cherish their time together. It's so important to grab these times now.

***

Fidelma and Pearse from the advertising agency have arrived and we're all gathered in Dad's apartment to watch the preview of the final two ads. The ads will be released in two weeks, airing on Ash Wednesday. They're hoping these ads will hit home with people who might be considering giving up cigarettes for Lent.

We're watching the ads here because Dad is too sick to go outside. A car journey of any sort is out of the question. Because he is so unwell he has been in bed all day, but he's managed to make it to his chair in the sitting room for the viewing. He is out of sorts because he's in pain, though, and it doesn't look like he has much energy to give. As a result, there's a slightly hurried feeling in the room to get the ads on quickly.

The room feels packed as we all sit or stand where we can. There's been a bit of an issue with getting the laptop going but it looks like it's just been fixed. 'Okay, guys, here we go, these are the next two ads,' Fidelma announces. 'The first one is called "Family" and the last one is called "Gratitude".' Then she turns and pulls the curtain, as there's a shine on the screen.

She presses play.

Silence.

We watch the first one.

It ends after thirty seconds.

And I am horrified.

Calm down, Lisa. Calm down.

I look around and scan the faces of everyone else. They're all smiling and nodding. *Oh no, this is not good.* They obviously don't see what I just saw. Or maybe they have but it doesn't seem *that* bad to them.

'That's great, Fidelma, well done,' says Paddy, smiling. There's more agreeable nodding from the others.

Oh no. They definitely haven't seen what I saw.

The ad has been done in such a way that it shows Dad talking about Ciara, Stephen and me. About how much he'll miss us and about how much he'll miss being there for us when he's gone. The footage shows the three of us separately and Dad's voice-over describing us individually. The ad had started with him depicting me.

Fidelma plays the second ad, which is about what Dad is grateful for and what he values about his life. This ad ends with a great line from Dad: 'Don't smoke, don't start, and for those who have, stop.'

But I don't hear it.

I nod and half smile as everyone is chatting away about how much they love the ads. I think my stress levels are too high for this. The first ad has the potential to tip me onto the wrong side of the scales. I need to leave.

I look at Dad. He's in a lot of pain now and is quite disgruntled. Did he see what I saw? He looks me straight in the eyes from across the room and nods. His face is very serious. I think he did. I think he saw what I saw.

Right, I have no idea what I'm going to do about this but I know now is not the time.

Everyone starts to get ready to leave and Mum helps Dad go back to bed.

***

I wake in the morning and the ad is still on my mind, so I call over to Dad. As I sit at the end of his bed and hand him a smoothie, he sits himself up further.

'How are you feeling?' I ask.

'Getting there. Just need to pick up a bit and then I'll be okay. How are you after watching the ads?'

'Yeah, good, Dad. The ads were absolutely brilliant. You did an amazing job. You're really going to make a difference with them. Nana looks great in the one she's in. It's so lovely, the two of you walking down Dún Laoghaire pier together and so nice that Mum got in on the act too! I knew she'd give in eventually!' I laugh.

'Well, it was great actually because we were doing a small bit of filming in Vincent's one day, she popped in to see how I was getting on and I somehow managed to get her to just walk beside me for a bit while filming. I think she was secretly happy.'

'Yeah, I think so. It was done so tastefully. Are you happy with them?'

'I am. They've done a great job. There's one bit I'm not happy with, though, and I don't think you are either.'

I was right; he had noticed it. In that ad where he talks about his children he depicts Stephen as having a blend of drive and discipline and Ciara as being the brains of the family. But the words that were chosen from Dad's interview to describe me were lacking in description a bit. They weren't wrong or bad, necessarily; they just didn't do justice to the relationship that Dad and I have. There was mention of my age, that I was the first-born and that I'm genuine. That was it, basically.

'Yeah, to be honest, I panicked when I saw it. It stood out like a sore thumb.'

'I totally agree,' Dad says. 'The thing was when we were filming we had no idea the exact route the ads would go down or what footage would be used for what in the end. It's also hard to think of everything on the spot.'

I know exactly what he means. My spotlight meltdown was a classic example. I could barely summon up one memory of us together, never mind describing my relationship with him. I have a feeling I will look back on this and wonder how the hell we all managed to do this.

'I'll ring Fidelma now and talk to her. Tell her we need to get even just a mic in here so I can record more. I'd like to do that,' he says.

'I can suggest some descriptive words for you to say,' I laugh. 'Lisa is just a fabulous girl altogether, hilarious and witty, not to mention the best person ever. Something along those lines, perhaps?'

He laughs but his laugh is weak. Very weak, I notice.

'I'll get on to Fidelma now.'

He picks up the phone and calls her.

Fidelma rings me shortly afterwards and, as soon as we talk

through everything, my stress levels decrease almost instantly. She understands implicitly the enormity of this situation and the need for this to feel right to both of us. If it's going to be on TV and in the ether for years to come, long after Dad goes, then it can't be wrong. It just can't be.

We decide the best thing to do is have the team take another stab at it.

Fidelma estimates that it will take today and possibly tomorrow to get the new draft completed. In fact it was to take a bit longer and other issues soon became more important.

***

Dad missed his Sunday session at The Hot Spot yesterday. It's the first one he's missed since all this started. Cancer or no cancer he has been there every week. Sunday last I was down there with him and it was clear that he wasn't feeling great. Looking back, he really shouldn't have been there, as he hadn't long finished his chemo session.

It's late in the afternoon when I notice a missed call on my phone. I must have left it on silent. It was Rosemary. I call her back.

'Hi, Rosemary, sorry I missed you!'

'Hi, Lisa.' She sounds a bit panicked. 'I'm here with your dad, and I just don't like how he is. I'm really worried. He has a temperature and he's not eating anything. He says he's fine but I really don't like it. He's been like this for a few days. It's just going on for too long now.'

I had only been thinking about this earlier. It's been over a week since Dad's gotten out of bed, bar the hour for watching the ads late last week. Is that not strange? Something is not adding up.

The palliative care nurses have been in and out and they are seeing to him regularly. They are trying different tablets to get his bowels moving for him but each time they try a different one we have to wait to see if there's any improvement. There seems to be a lot of waiting.

He has not pulled up at all from the chemo session. Why not? The cycle of the chemo should have passed by now, come to think of it, and he should be feeling on the better side of things.

'I'll call over to you now, Rosemary.'

I'm a bit nervous as I run across the road. Once inside the apartment, I go straight to Dad's bedroom.

'Hi, Dad, you still not feeling better you poor thing?'

I've a smile on my face so as not to let him see that I'm worried. He's still lying in bed and he looks very pale and I think he's lost more weight since yesterday, if that's even possible.

'Hi, honey. Yeah I'm like a frustrated mathematician here, still trying to work it out,' he jokes. He's so good at trying to make things easier on everyone else.

He definitely has a temperature so we decide to ring the doctor. Perhaps he has an infection and that's what's keeping him sick. He may need antibiotics to help him fight it off.

Rosemary looks very shaken and I feel it too. We ring the doctor and leave Dad to rest. Afterwards, we have tea in the kitchen and both cry. It's so hard to watch the person you love lie in bed, in pain, unable to get up and do the things he wants to do. He hasn't been able to box since December; he hasn't been able to pick up the guitar in a couple of weeks. These things are like oxygen to him and not being able to do them is detrimental to his soul.

The doctor arrives in about an hour and we all go back in to Dad. I have to say, at the time, in my eyes this doctor is pretty crap. Having discussed Dad's history, he says there's probably not a whole lot he can do for him. Dad seems fine with that prognosis but I am absolutely not.

'Well if there's nothing you can do, should you not send him into the hospital? An IV drip with fluids and vitamins would be a good start don't you think? The man hasn't been able to eat or get much into him, as you know.'

What a moron, I think. *Why am I the one who is having to think of things he can do? I am doing his job for him.*

His response to this suggestion seems even more ridiculous. He says Dad won't benefit much by going to the hospital.

Dad is nodding his head, saying he'll be fine. He even thanks the doctor for calling in! I don't get it! This is so frustrating. So much for being a health-care physician. I'd say he couldn't take care of a goldfish. (In hindsight I can admit I was too hard on this doctor – he clearly realised that Dad was in a much worse way by then than I was willing to accept and there was little he could have done for him at this stage.)

'Can't you even prescribe him some Ensures to drink?' I ask, my hands in the air, wearing my rage like armour.

Ensures are protein drinks for people who can't get food into them. They're not like having a tasty steak but they're not awful either. In fact, I could probably do with a few of them myself. Can't say I've been eating much these last couple of months. Instead, constant anxiety tends to fill up my stomach, leaving no room for food.

Dad agrees that Ensures are the way forward and the doctor gets out his pen and pad and writes a prescription. Then he shakes Dad's hand and leaves.

'Okay, Dad, let's get some Ensures into you today then and see how you feel tomorrow,' I tell him.

I head off to fill the prescription and then return with the Ensures to the apartment. I give Dad a vanilla one and he sips away on that. Rosemary puts the rest of them in the fridge.

I sit down on the bed beside him and I can feel all the tears I've been holding back all morning gathering behind my eyes. I am flicking through a magazine, not reading any of it. I just want to be beside him for a bit.

'You okay, hun?'

I glance at him. He looks so sick. I am so angry inside my head: *Why can't he just get better? Why? Just fix the problem, medical people, and make his body work properly again! Please!*

Aloud, I say: 'I just want you to feel better Dad. This is so shit for you.' He nods and passes me a tissue.

***

The next day a family meeting is called with the palliative care people. We all meet in Dad's apartment. From the family, there's me, Mum, Stephen, Paddy, Declan and Rosemary. Ciara is away in New York; she's due back in a couple of days. Dad is in bed with the door closed and we are all in the sitting room.

When I arrive there's an older woman I don't recognise with one of the care nurses I do recognise. The older lady is probably in her late fifties. She has a friendly face. Paddy arrives in last and, once he is seated, we begin.

The woman introduces herself; she's from Blackrock Hospice and explains that she works alongside and oversees the palliative care team. She explains that she has already been in with Dad and had a look at him. She feels that he is not pulling up at the moment and that he needs help with his pain management. Consequently, she thinks that some respite in the hospice will help get him back on track.

Respite? I've heard this term before but I've never needed to know exactly what it means. I suddenly feel fortunate that this is my first encounter with it.

'He can just go in for a few days until he feels better and things are flowing as they should be, then he can come back home,' she assures us.

I'm watching the others to see how they are receiving this news, as I'm not entirely sure what to make of it. Some of them look upset, while the rest seem confident that this is a good thing. I think this is a good thing. I think. I know she said *hospice* but if they can help get him back on track I'm all for it. I actually feel a sense of relief. At least there are some capable people here telling us they can help him. This woman seems to know her stuff.

Once we're all in agreement that this is the right step to help

Dad, she says she'll go in and talk with him and explain to him what happens next. I feel a bit like a deer caught in headlights, even though I'm in agreement with this plan.

She goes in to Dad, and Mum and Rosemary go with her. He'll be going in tomorrow morning, it seems. *Good*, I think. The sooner he goes in the sooner he'll get out.

17

THE HOSPICE

'I don't know if I'm getting out of here, lads.' Dad is not smiling as he says this. In fact, he is in a lot of pain right now.

Mum and I are helping ease him back into his bed from a trip to the bathroom. All our movements are awkward. I suspect that, despite our best intentions, he'd rather not have us help him like this. But unfortunately there's nothing we can do about it. He needs us. In an effort to ease his discomfort, I avert my eyes as much as possible.

'Of course you are, Dad,' I say. 'You're literally going to be here for a few days while they get your pain levels under control, then you'll be back in business and back in your own place.'

'You've got Glengarriff to get to, don't forget,' Mum chimes in.

His statement has caught me totally off guard. He never says things as defeatist as that, unless they're followed swiftly by some optimistic saying or positive projection. My response also seemed a little off, a bit empty or something. Why is that? I do believe what I just said. Until yesterday I thought hospices were for people who are about to die but now I know people also come in for pain management and respite. That's good. I'm glad he's here. Right?

Mum and I get him settled, make sure his drip is okay. He has his lip-balm within reach and has water to hand. He hates when his lips are dry. I look around the room, noting how clean, spacious and minimalistic it is. There are two French doors leading outside to a patio. They are letting welcome light through, filling the room and adding a sense of peace to the scene. It's very quiet here. I like that. I know Dad does too. The bed he's in is wide, which is great because there's no risk of him falling out. However, he's a tall man and it seems only just long enough for him. It reminds me of a super version of a hospital trolley; it has those steel sidebars that can be pulled up or let down and it's also on wheels, but it looks much bigger and more comfy.

Dad falls asleep in seconds. He's so tired all the time. Mum and I decide to go for a wander. She fills me in on the earlier events of the day as we walk. By all accounts getting Dad from his apartment to the hospice was a traumatic experience. Mum and Declan brought him in. Thank God Declan was there to help because he is the only one big and strong enough to hold Dad up. As I listen to Mum tell me how things went, I am actually so glad I wasn't there. Is that bad? I just don't know if I could bear to see him in so much agony. He is so weak right now, in so much pain that any movement is agonising for him.

We make our way to the cafeteria we both saw on our way in, go up to the counter and order tea. Neither of us feels hungry, though we get a couple of Snack bars to go with our tea. The cafeteria is pretty sizable. The roof is made mostly of glass panels. I'm sensing a general trend for light throughout the building. There's no one else in here. It appears we caught the café just before it closes.

Mum looks tired and a bit shaken. Florence Nightingale, Dad always calls her. She's a carer by nature, which is a beautiful way to be. She always knows what to do and how to do it. I wish I could be more like her in that regard. I'm not saying I'm selfish, but sometimes I don't help in the practical ways that she does. Maybe that comes down to experience? All that said, this is definitely taking its toll on her. She looks way older than she is at the moment and I can see strong lines cutting through finer lines under both eyes. They weren't there before. Or, if they were, they certainly weren't as severe. Worry runs deep, it appears.

After a while, I decide to investigate the place. It really is so quiet here but there's a nice feeling about it. I didn't expect that. I've never been to a hospice, so I had no idea what to expect, but in my mind I was thinking of something like an old folks home, one that's rundown and smelly and sad. This is bright and clean, and the receptionist is really nice. It's strange being in a place that is purpose-built for people to leave this world. How many souls have left from this building, I wonder?

Around the corner of the cafeteria and down the hall I come across the entrance to a small chapel. Inside, there are pews and an altar and a small organ that looks not unlike a full-sized keyboard. I'm not religious but I appreciate why people would come here: to seek solace, to find time for themselves and try to find peace. I imagine a lot of people might attempt to make deals with God in here. *I will do this, if you save my person.* I am tempted to do this. It's a funny time. I do find myself wondering about God a lot. How that one word has such different meanings to different people throughout the entire world. It has brought peace and safety to many, and pain and suffering to many others. I wonder about my own beliefs. I wonder about all the millions of beliefs in the world. Are any of us right? Will we actually ever find out? If you got it wrong do you get another go? Something that has run through my mind from time to time over the years is whether I, in the face of losing a member of my tribe, would jump ship back to Catholicism. Just in case I'd got it wrong.

I haven't so far, anyway.

I walk slowly back up the corridor. There aren't many rooms, roughly twelve. We were very lucky to get Dad in here. I peer into the rooms discreetly as I pass. From what I can see they are all similar to Dad's room. I see some family members in with their person. The scene in one room in particular strikes my heart. There's an elderly woman crying as she holds the hand of the person in bed. Due to the angle, I cannot see the person's face but their aged hands tell me their story. Man and wife. Lived through decades together. Love. Hardship. Friends. Memories. Probably kids. One is leaving now and they are both heartbroken from the impending loss.

I sit down on a bench opposite Dad's room. The door to his room is open and all I can see are his feet sticking out over the end of the bed. I can't go in just yet. I just continue to stare at his feet. They are such big feet. It's ridiculous. No wonder they never have his size in the shops. I feel a bit strange right now. There's a feeling of something coming together or coming apart; I'm not entirely sure which one it is. As I continue to stare, my mind starts to wonder how long I will keep getting to see his feet in that bed. Is he really about to leave us forever? It's so painful to imagine what life will be like without him.

Crap. Tears are streaming down my face again. Note to self: for the love of God buy some nice balm tissues for yourself. You've enough to be dealing with without having a chapped, dry nose. I go to the loo and use the almost paper-like tissue. I try to compose myself before I head back out.

***

I'm back home when Fidelma gets back to me with the revised version of the ad. Unfortunately the panic kicks back in. I watch it three times to make absolutely certain. It's still not right. What am I supposed to do here? Dad is now in the hospice and I'm here trying to get this right. I feel so all at sea.

After a few moments of sitting and trying my best to meditate, I know exactly what I need to do. I need to go to the source. I need to talk to Steph. She's gone back to LA but I can still get in touch. She was there with him in the trenches. Interviewing him. The others weren't there so it's hard for them to piece this together. She is my last hope to get this right. I get out my laptop and send her an email explaining where I'm at with this.

Steph calls me literally within hours, sounding concerned. 'Hi, Lisa, are you okay?' she starts. 'I am fully up to speed with everything.' Steph is ridiculously efficient. I know she is currently directing a movie and there's a lot going on for her, so I really appreciate her time and effort.

'Thanks so much for calling, Steph. I know you are probably knee deep in *Run and Jump* right now, but I really feel you might be able to help with this. You were the one who was right there beside him throughout.'

'No problem at all. I'm really happy you reached out and that I can work with you on this. Fidelma and I spoke at length and we both agree the obvious answer to the situation, in an ideal world, is that we would get the crew back into your dad's place for an hour, he would say what he wants to say and the guys would just film it in the same fashion as last time. But that's not an option now. Aside from the fact that he is not physically well enough to sit up, his vocal chords have weakened, so his voice would sound dramatically different to the other parts of the ad. That leaves us with option B, which is you going back over all the footage they already have from the interviews with your dad.'

They read my mind.

Steph continues. 'Fidelma is sending you through all the footage, and giving you some alternative words and phrases your Dad used when describing your relationship and his thoughts about you in a word document, in an effort to help you see things clearly. Fidelma's team has already been briefed and is aware of the situation. She tells me they are just as determined as we are to get it right.'

Time is of the essence, so I immediately sit down at my sitting-room table, open my email with the word document attached, download the footage and start watching. Jesus, it's hard to watch. But I know that now is no time for emotion. This has to be done as quickly as possible.

I watch the three-minute footage. Immediately there is one sentence that sticks out to me. It refers more to how I was back in my late teens/early twenties, but it's as real as real can be: 'Lisa was the rebellious one. She was the one that would put the phone down telling you she wasn't coming home.'

I watch him say that sentence and give a long, loud belly laugh. He goes on to tell them stories about my trying teenage years and continues laughing as he recalls my numerous rebellions. I know why he's laughing; it's because I remind him of how he was at that age. At the time I was without doubt a pain in the ass but, upon reflection, I know he loved that I just did my own thing regardless of what he said.

Right, that has to go in.

I put that in place in the word document and swap the second and third sentence with each other. The rest is fine. I move a couple of screenshots to flow slightly better with the new sequence and that's it.

There. It's done. It's as close to how I think he would want it to be as I can get it. I send back all the directions to Fidelma and she liaises with the editing team to get started on the revisions. I follow up with Steph and she is delighted that it's now as I need it to be.

I let out the biggest breath. *Thank God.* It shouldn't take long; the team is on standby.

***

I arrive in to Dad that evening with the new version of the ad on my laptop ready for viewing. I knock gently and walk into his room. He's slightly elevated in the bed and half asleep.

'Hi, Dad,' I say gently.

He perks up as I lean in for a hug. Then he pushes me away, looking completely repulsed. 'Lisa,' he cries.

What now? I definitely don't have any perfume on! Oh crap. Yes. I completely forgot about my cold sore. In fact, it's gone from one mildly mannered one on my top lip yesterday to three outrageously angry ones today. I should probably have a warning bell around my neck. Dad is clearly horrified I even attempted to give him a hug.

'Ah, Dad. Sure you've more to be worried about than a few cold sores at this stage!' I joke.

We both laugh. I'm not wrong. We laugh even harder. About the cut of me, the cut of him – the cut of the whole damn situation.

'Right, it's sorted,' I tell him. 'I have the new ad. Are you up to seeing it?' I'm keeping my voice low, as he's a bit drowsy.

'Absolutely,' he says, trying to sit up.

I help him, and then I put the laptop on his lap and sit down in the chair beside him.

He presses play.

'Lisa was rebellious. I love being in her company, she's 100% genuine. Stephen's got the blend of the drive and the discipline. Ciara's the brains of the family, and she has a heart of gold.'

As he watches the ad, I watch him.

When it finishes he looks over at me.

'Perfect,' he says. I can see the relief and happiness in his eyes. 'I couldn't have said it better myself.'

The tiredness is upon him instantly. I put the laptop down and help him back to a lying position and hand him his mouth gel. 'I need to get some sleep now, honey. Well done to everyone again. I'm so happy.'

I turn off the main light and leave his side lamp on for him. I look around and am glad to see his room looking homely. We had brought in family photos and his guitar just to help with that sense of familiarity.

He closes his eyes and is asleep before I leave the room. I hope he feels better tomorrow.

MARCH 2014

18

WE NEED TO TALK ABOUT GERRY

There has been a lot of hanging around in here.

Dad is asleep almost all of the time now. I'm spending a lot of time in the cafeteria. People are in the room with him frequently, keeping him company and chatting while he's awake. I'm not. I'm finding it too hard. I go in and all I want to do is cry. It's not fair for Dad to see me like this. It's hard enough on him as it is. If I'm finding this excruciating, imagine what he must be feeling. People crying at him is not what he needs right now. Plus I just can't seem to find the right words to say. It's the oddest thing. Never, in my whole life, have I struggled to find words to say to Dad. Yet now, when he might need me most, I'm out having tea in the cafeteria.

As I finish off my drink, Ciara comes in and says that Ursula wants to have a conversation with the family. Ursula is the psychologist at the hospice. Okay. I instantly feel a stupid giddy feeling coming on and a surge of energy running up and down my body. I really want her to say that things are looking up but I sense that might not be the case. Either way, Stephen's not here so we should probably hold on until he arrives.

'Stephen's not here but she says she'll talk to him later,' Ciara says, as if reading my mind.

I follow Ciara down to a room that's in the same end of the building as Dad's. Mum is in there already on her own, waiting for us. She smiles at us when we walk in. She has a softness to her that is comforting.

This giddy feeling is really taking over and I can feel sparks flying around my body. I shake my arms, trying to get rid of the nervous energy. We all sit on the couch. Mum is beside me, and Ciara beside her. The room is fairly standard. There are a few ladies magazines on the glass coffee table and some toys in the corner for kids to play with it. That's it.

Ursula walks in. I met her briefly before. Her face is oval, her complexion is great and her skin has a nice warm colour. She has friendly eyes; they're a nice hazel colour, which gives them a warmth. Her hair is pulled back from her face in a professional manner. She sits in front of us and introduces herself again. She engages full eye contact with each of us one after the other. I like that.

'So, as you know, when we brought Gerry in here five days ago, it was to help with the pain he's in and to get it under control to the point where he can go back home.'

We agree with nods and hums.

'Since then we've monitored him very closely and watched his condition microscopically.'

More nodding from us.

'It's at this point that I have to be honest with you. We are not happy with Gerry's progression and in fact he has gotten worse.'

Pause.

'A lot worse, unfortunately.'

I want to laugh. I think she's about to tell us the sort of news I've seen people on *ER* get. I cannot believe this is happening. My mind goes into overdrive. He is not going to die. He's my dad. He is invincible. This all has to be a big joke. How the hell have the last few months been so insane? Right, if she doesn't say the word die or dead in her next sentence then I reckon the coast is clear. Do they not know Ciara is only twenty-five? She can't lose her dad at this age; he hasn't even gotten to make a nice speech at her thirtieth like he did at mine. Nope. It's too soon for this. He's too young. We're all too bloody young!

'We usually gauge people on how well they are doing day by day and that's generally how we can tell how long it will be before we can let them home. The sad thing is that Gerry has been slipping in the other direction and we feel that he is leaving us.'

Fuck.

'When a person is going in *that* direction we generally gauge how long they have left by how fast they are deteriorating. If they are deteriorating at a rate of months then they usually still have months left. If they are deteriorating by weeks then they have weeks left. If they are deteriorating by days then they more than likely have days left.'

Pause. I feel really light-headed. My mouth has gone totally dry.

Ursula tilts her head slightly, purses her lips and drops her eyes for a minute before looking back up and directly at us.

'I'm really sorry to have to say this but Gerry appears to be deteriorating by days and hours at this point. I think it's time to call the family in and let people know that Gerry is dying now.'

There it is. *Dying.* She has done her job.

I breathe in slowly through my nose and fill my lungs with air and hold it. I can feel the rage inside me starting but it dies down quickly. There's no more resistance. I know.

I exhale. As I let the air out of my lungs, any denial that had crept back in over the last week – protecting me from what I couldn't deal with – is released. This is happening. And it's happening right now.

None of us move. We are just staring at her. I reach for some water I had brought in with me. I can't speak.

'Gerry knows. We spoke to him just before talking to you. He's taking some time to digest the news. He wanted me to tell you on your own, without him there, so you can also digest the news and be free in yourselves.'

A massive lump is growing in my throat. It hurts like hell. He wanted us to be able to cry. Bless him. Why is *he* dying? There are horrible people in the world, who just hurt others and who live for far too long, and here's Dad, such a great person, dying and he's only fifty-seven!

'I'm going to leave you now and give you some time to process everything. You might want to ring Stephen and tell him to leave work now and come here.'

What? Oh my God. This is truly happening now. He can't

even wait to finish work? This is all too much. The adrenaline is surging through my veins. I need to laugh or cry or burst into some crazy dance.

We thank Ursula and she leaves. Mum hugs us both. Ciara breaks down and looks absolutely horrified as the news filters through. I can literally see her heart breaking through her eyes. I wish this didn't have to happen to her.

After a few minutes Mum goes to ring Stephen. Ciara and I stand outside the room. We are silent and still in shock.

'Get in,' I say, pointing at an empty wheelchair. Without hesitation Ciara jumps in and before we know it I am pushing her up the corridor and we are gaining speed. She is laughing hysterically because it's totally inappropriate and getting borderline dangerous now. I see a small turn to the right coming up. It leads to a smaller corridor that ends with a glass door to the outside. I lean a hard right, the chair turns relatively easily and down we go. We come to a sudden halt inches away from the door. I try to back up and do a three-point turn but it's too tight and I have no idea what I'm doing. Ciara jumps out and again we burst into laughter. We are laughing so hard we can barely breathe. I have to sit on the floor and hold my stomach. Tears are streaming down both our faces.

Declan arrives down and we see him passing. He doesn't see us. Declan is my godfather and I love him to bits.

'Declan!'

We go after him. He turns. He's crying. He's obviously just gotten the news. He looks like a little boy. Dad is his big brother and this must be so hard for him. I can't imagine what it must be like, getting the news that your sibling is about to die.

Declan gives us both a hug. As the three of us stand there and embrace, Ciara and I start laughing simultaneously. We are obviously both thinking the same thing.

'What?' says Declan.

'Oh, you are *so* going to be hounded for dad hugs,' laughs Ciara.

'Oh absolutely. You are exactly the same as Dad,' I chime in.

This thought lifts the mood slightly and there's a lovely sense of family and love now. I bask in this feeling for as long as I can.

***

Mum comes and gets Ciara and me from the cafeteria. Stephen has arrived and has been told. Dad has called all four of us to his room.

'Well, lads, this is it,' Dad says as we enter. 'The last minute of the match.'

We're all standing around Dad's bed. Mum, Stephen, Ciara and I. I'm at the foot of the bed with Mum just to the left of me, Stephen is standing beside Dad on the right-hand side of the bed holding his hand, with Ciara on the other side. She looks pale and absolutely distraught.

I have no words. I don't know what to say. I actually feel oddly numb in my body.

'I couldn't be more proud of you all. I'm ready, guys.' His words are like sweet daggers in my heart. I can't describe how much I love this man. I can't believe he's actually leaving me here. People say you'll never know love until you have a child.

Well, I say to them, you'll never know love until you've had a Gerry Collins as your dad.

Suddenly Stephen breaks down crying and puts his free hand to his head, trying to cover his face. Oh God. This is the saddest thing I've ever seen. I haven't seen Stephen cry once through this whole thing. Jesus. This is devastating.

Dad reaches up with his other hand and pulls Stephen down to him into an embrace. He holds Stephen to him. Stephen is just sobbing and sobbing. My heart is going to full on smash into tiny particles right now. *Do. Not. Cry. Lisa.* Be brave. This is their moment. Be strong and let them cry together without having to think of comforting anyone else.

'Come here, Steve. You're a great man. I love you very much.'

Stephen, a few minutes later, stands upright again and wipes his face with his sleeve. Mum throws him over a Kleenex. How does she always have tissues to hand exactly when someone needs them?

I'm starting to panic. I still can't seem to grasp the right words to say. I've been trying to write something for the last few days so I can read it out to him or even let him read it in his own time but the words just will not come. All the things I tried to write seemed so lame. The likes of 'I love you' just sounds so generic and obvious. He knows how much I love him. I feel I need to say something but here, in the moment, sweet Jesus, there are no words. Please words, come. Time is truly not on our side here.

'I'll say something at your funeral, Dad,' I suddenly blurt out.

He looks at me. 'Will you, Lisa?' He's smiling but also looks a bit surprised. I have to say I'm a bit surprised myself. That's not exactly what I had in mind. My fear of public speaking is well known. But now that I've said it I know it's something I actually have to do. And I want him to know I'm going to do it. A gesture. To show him my love for him is bigger than my fear of public speaking. That says a lot.

'Well, wouldn't that be lovely. I would really love that,' he says.

I smile back and nod. I'm afraid if I say anything else I will fully dissolve into a river of tears. I don't even have anything else to say.

'Dad NO, you can *still* beat this,' cries Ciara. She looks utterly traumatised, like she's in a horror movie. When I look at her I see someone trying to empty a sinking boat with her hands. The damage to the boat is too severe and she knows it, but she refuses to give up. She is exhausted yet completely unrelenting.

Dad looks at her and reaches out to her.

'Come here, pet. I know this is so hard but this is happening now, honey.'

Ciara drops her head and tears are dropping to the ground.

'No,' she whispers. 'No.'

Dad pulls her closer to him. She resists, as if giving in to his hug means she has lost the war.

'Come here.' Dad tugs her down to him and she bawls into his chest.

Honestly, I feel like I'm out of my body right now. I am somewhere floating above, watching it all yet wanting to look away. My little human brain is about to explode.

I look at Mum. She's standing slightly back with silent tears streaming down her face.

Ciara stands up again and tries to compose herself. I meet her eyes. By way of a nod I let her know I'm here for her.

After a few minutes, Stephen, Ciara and I leave Mum to talk with Dad on her own. I look back and see Mum pull up a chair and hold Dad's hand. She leans in to him, as if to lie by him for a while, his hand on her face. To so clearly see their love for each other, after all these years and everything they've gone through, is without doubt the most beautiful thing I have ever seen.

19

GOODBYE DAD

Dad received a letter from the Minister of Health yesterday. Dr Fenton Howell, whom I met so many months ago, hand-delivered it to the hospice that evening. There was great excitement and sense of achievement when we opened it. In it, he thanked Dad for his contribution to the campaign and said how his story will 'help the wellbeing of our population'. Well now, if that isn't something to be proud of, I don't know what is. It's a pity Dad hasn't woken up to see it. He hasn't woken up since yesterday morning. Paddy read it to him, so hopefully he heard it.

Becki stayed upstairs in the hospice with me last night. I'm so thankful she is here. Mum and Ciara stayed down with Dad in his room. Ciara was adamant about not leaving him on his own overnight, so they both slept in lazy-boy chairs.

Friends of Dad's have wanted to come in and see him these past few days but at this stage only family members are allowed to see him. The nurses have mentioned to us that Dad now needs quiet. Even though he's asleep he will be distracted by noise and by the chatter of people around his bed. They have asked if people do need to see him that they be very mindful that he is dying. Have you ever tried to go to sleep and couldn't? And when, finally, you are on the brink of nodding off, someone downstairs starts talking loudly and it pulls you right back out of wherever you are and back to being awake but completely agitated? Well that's where Dad is right now. He's got one foot in this world and one in another so he needs quiet to make the transition.

I have to say, I've never actually been under such pressure. I feel like we're all in a car crash advert on TV. One where the camera is showing the road from the driver's viewpoint and we can hear the music singing sweetly as he's driving, but we know what's coming. We're bracing ourselves, hoping and wishing somehow that the crash won't happen but we know it will and any moment now the chaos and devastation will be unleashed.

I'm currently having tea in the cafeteria, relaxing in that very moment. Chatting to Paddy. I am listening to him but I'm also aware that I look like I got dragged through a bush backwards. I just didn't have time to pack and bring clean clothes. Kat dropped some stuff in to me yesterday, which was great, but I forgot to ask for loads of things, including my make-up.

Paddy's chatting away about anything. He's great. But out of nowhere I feel an overwhelming urge to talk to Dad. I'm sitting here trying to figure out what is causing this. Then it hits me like a train. I know what I need to say to him!

'Sorry, Paddy!' I say suddenly and jump up. 'I have to go down to Dad.'

Oh God. The panic inside me is unreal. Finally I know what it is I need to tell him. I just have to say this to him and quickly!

I run full speed down the corridor. I get to his door and stop for a second outside, then push open the door quietly.

'Oh, hi, Mum, hi, Cathy.' Mum and her sister Cathy are here. Damn. They need to leave.

'Mum, can I have a minute with Dad, please?'

I'm trying to stay calm but I am freaking out inside.

'Sure.'

They leave and I am just willing them to move faster. Hurry up, hurry up. They close the door slowly. Come on!

Oh Jesus.

'Dad.' I stand by his right-hand side and hold his hand. 'Dad, it's me. I know what I need to tell you now.' I'm whispering. I don't want to disturb him but I need to say this loud enough so he hears me. I stand in closer. It's so obvious. How did I not think to say this to him before now? We have all been so worried about him but that isn't *his* concern.

'I hear you've been worrying about us. But listen to me now and listen well, you *do not* have to worry about us. Do you hear me? We have so much of your blood running through our veins and that will get us through anything. We have amazing people around us and we have each other. You do not have anything to worry about.' Tears are streaming down my face. 'We are all here for you. You have been an amazing Dad and thank you so much for everything. I love you so much.'

Suddenly there's a stop in his breathing. I lift my head quickly. Is it just a gap? My eyes go wide and wild. Oh Jesus.

Oh Jesus. He's not breathing. His breathing has been shallow and with long pauses but I think this is too long.

I hold his hand tighter. Shit, there's no one here. I don't know what to do. I can't leave him in this moment.

Suddenly Ciara comes into the room.

'Ciara! I think he's dying!' I say. 'Where's the bell?'

She gasps and runs to the other side of the bed where the emergency button is. She grabs his other hand and presses the bell.

There's another shallow gasp for breath from Dad. We go utterly still. Staring ferociously at him. Is this really it?

The nurses come in.

'We think he's dying!'

They jump into action. One turns and leaves the room and the other moves swiftly to the top of his bed and checks something.

Oh God. He's leaving. I can feel it.

All of a sudden everyone appears around his bed. The other nurse must have got them. Phew. I can hear their cries and their goodbyes as they all huddle closely around us. I close my eyes and drop to the ground and sit cross-legged in a seated position. His hand still in my hands, I rest my forehead on it. Everyone else starts to melt into the background and I can no longer hear them. I just want this moment to last for as long as possible, and for it to be private. I close my eyes harder and I feel like I'm in a little cocoon – one that contains just Dad and me. His hand is warm but starting to radiate heat. I instinctively know what it is. It's him and he's getting ready. His energy is starting to move. I know it. I've never felt anything like it before but I know exactly what's happening.

There's no question. The heat is slowly starting to move around my hand and down my arm and in seconds I feel completely surrounded by it. Suddenly I feel really calm. I feel like I'm suspended in time and I am not one bit sad. In fact, I feel joy and peace. I feel like I'm getting a glimpse into the future and that I'm going to be okay. There was a time I thought I'd have to throw myself on top of Dad's grave if he were ever to die before me. Yet here I am, holding his hand as he dies, and I feel okay. I'm going to be okay. We are all going to be okay because he'll be around; it'll just be in a different way. I want to stay here in this cocoon forever, it's so peaceful.

Then, slowly, the heat starts to leave me. *Oh no! Please stay!* I can feel the dread and devastation as reality floods in and I tune back into the room. I hear the cries. Their cries. My cries. It's gone. He's gone. He has left his body. His hand is cold. I still hold it to me.

But I know now. He's shown me.

We are going to be okay. Maybe not straightaway. But without doubt, in time, we will all feel joy once again.

EPILOGUE

'I'm telling you, honey, I know everyone is worried but this is going to be a good thing. I promise.'

Gerry Collins

We had no idea when we started this journey what was ahead of us all. We had no clue of the media frenzy that was going to surround Dad's story and the reach it would have throughout our country. We had no idea how much it would impact, not only the health policy in Ireland as we knew it then in 2014, but also directly the daily lives of over 175,000 Irish people. That Dad's own words would be quoted in Irish legislation standardising cigarette packaging, and he and the campaign would be referenced in the European Parliament as having created one of the most effective and powerful campaigns the EU has ever seen.

Dad was the only person who was certain of anything at the very beginning of this process. He was certain of three things:

1. That doing these ads would create good energy for him and our inner circle at a time when positivity would be hard to find.

2. That there was a lesson to his story. And that the road he had already gone down was one he'd like to save others from, if he could.

3. That doing this would bring his family closer together at a time when we would need each other.

He wasn't wrong.

After Dad died we were inundated with texts, emails and Facebook messages from people we knew, half knew, used to know or had never met. These were messages of condolence and sympathy, often coupled with stories of similar losses. It was a privilege to hear these stories. In many of them there was a sense of gratitude towards Dad, as he appeared to have either helped the person directly, or a family member, to stop smoking. The sense of a newfound hope for life wove its way through these emails. It was unbelievable.

A gentleman, from Limerick I believe, wrote to me one day. He shared with me his sympathies for my loss and told me about how his mum had died from cancer a few years back. He finished his message with something that has always stuck with me: 'I'm so sorry again for your loss but I'm sure the pride helps with the pain.'

He couldn't have been more right. It really has helped.

All I wanted to do for a long time after Dad died was talk about him with anyone who'd listen; with people who knew him and knew how much he meant to me, but also with people who didn't actually know him at all. However, I reckoned there would be a good chance, if I got his name in, that they might know who I was talking about. I couldn't help myself sometimes.

Here's a classic example. I remember one day, around ten months after Dad died, I was flying to Kuwait to meet my then boyfriend (now husband), Tiernan. Funnily enough, we had met through the campaign. Did Dad send him my way? Maybe he did, but that's another story. Tiernan was living in the Middle East at the time and so we were in a long-distance relationship, which meant travelling to meet each other a lot.

I was settling into my window seat on the Emirates flight en route to Kuwait, ready for the eight hours ahead. I was wearing my oversized travel hoodie that I love to fly in. I was just sitting there, and I was in a terrible mood as I found myself desperately missing Dad. The grief was colossal, as it had been for so much of that first year. But there was also something about being on a plane that deepened the grief. Probably it had something to do with being crammed into a small space with nowhere to go but into your head. Not a pretty place to be when you're in the depths of despair.

After a few minutes, a painfully happy couple in their late fifties filled the two empty seats beside me. *Oh, good God no.* I could overhear that they were going on to Dubai to celebrate their ten-year anniversary. I could tell from the lovely lilt in their accent that they were from Cork. When they sat down and had settled themselves I could feel them trying to catch my eye to say hello and welcome me into their world of cheeriness. *Sorry folks, NOT going to happen. You are FAR too happy for me to tolerate right now.* Up went my hood, to cover my face from them as much as I could. Earphones were immediately put in, arms were folded and that was the end of that.

I watched two movies and cried silently to myself.

Out of nowhere, four hours later, I felt a bit better. Something shifted in me and I felt like saying hi. Out came the earphones, the hood came down, the arms unfolded and I slightly angled myself their way.

'Hi,' I said with a smile on my face.

'Well, hello there,' said the lady sitting beside me. She had a lovely warm way about her. I instantly liked her vibe.

That was that. The barricade was down and I had a glass of champagne to join them in their celebrations. They told me that they were from Cork and then they explained what lay ahead of them for their week's holidays. Then, in true Irish style, the conversation came back to what we all do for a living, and the woman proceeded to tell me she was an oncology nurse in Cork University Hospital.

Well. An oncology nurse, you say? She was practically begging me to tell her about my dad. So I forced his story into the conversation with as much subtlety as a sledgehammer.

Once I'd finished telling them pretty much everything – though I didn't mention his name – they both put down their glasses and stared at me in silence. Looking back now, I know that I was being awkward and a bit of a downer. It just really helped me to talk about him. It was like I reconnected with him every time he was mentioned.

'Oh my God, Gerry is your dad?' exclaimed the man, looking a bit shocked.

Equally shocked, I looked back at him. I didn't expect them to know who I was talking about, never mind know my dad's name.

But here I was, on an Emirates flight to Kuwait, and a couple from Cork were shaking my hand and saying thank you to me in place of my dad for what he'd done for the health of the Irish people. It was just the most bizarre and pride-filled moment. I'll never forget it.

I guess maybe that's part of the reason why I started to write this book. I wasn't ready to let him go and I really wanted to encapsulate everything he had achieved in his final eight months. It truly was an extraordinary effort from an extraordinary man.

Another reason was probably because it had to come out – the grief was making me unwell. A year on from Dad's passing I was still very broken. But then something happened. Tiernan and I moved to Los Angeles for four months and it was there that I wrote this book. It came spilling out. I cried from my soul as I brought back up the trauma of losing Dad. But all these words needed to come out to clear a path to recovery. And now, four years on, I can say that although I am not the same, I have stopped crying and I have laughed lots in more recent times.

I remember when I did my first Wax It Studio Facebook post, years ago now, my dad sat with me reading and re-reading my launching post before I finally hit the 'post' button. That seemed like such a big deal at the time. Now I'm here, getting ready to 'post' this book out into the world and he's not here to check and make sure that it's right.

I can only hope that it is, and that it does justice to the extraordinary man that I knew. Gerry Collins. My dad.

FAMILY NOTES

Dad's death had a profound effect on our entire family, but so did the kindness shown to us by friends and family throughout the months from his diagnosis to his death. None of us will ever forget that, nor will we ever forget the pride with which Dad's Quit campaign filled us. Here, Mum, Ciara and Stephen share a few thoughts on the man we all loved so deeply and the impact he had.

DELLY

First, I would like to take the opportunity to thank some of the people who really made a difference to our family during Gerry's illness.

Thanks to Greystones Cancer Support, who supported us through Gerry's illness.

Thanks to the staff of St Vincent's University Hospital, where Gerry received such wonderful care.

Thanks also to the palliative care team at Blackrock Hospice, especially for the support they gave us during and after Gerry's death.

And a huge thanks for all the support from family and friends, who were always there when we needed them.

To Gerry himself I would like to say, what a journey we travelled together over the last thirty-five years. It was amazing and I'm so grateful to have had that time with you. We were blessed to have three fabulous children. You also have two grandchildren now: Noah, who you met, and Sienna, who is eight months old. Noah still talks about his Gang Gang and him being up in the sky! Your name is often mentioned in the house and you are greatly missed by all of us.

The day you talked to me about your idea to do the ad I just knew it was going to happen, even though I was worried about the impact it would have on all the family. Your enthusiasm was next to none and wild horses couldn't have stopped you. But I honestly never thought for a minute that it would have the impact it did. Gerry, you and the kids did great. I'm so proud of you and how brave you were right up to the end. I know you are so proud of each one of the kids, as am I, particularly where they are in their lives today, and I know you are smiling down on them.

Gerry I miss you and will see you for a dance 'on the bright side of the road'.

Finally, I would like to express how proud I am of Lisa for putting this book together, and want to thank her from the bottom of my heart for all the hard work she has put into it.

CIARA

'If at least one person stops smoking because of this campaign then it will be worth it.'

These were the genuine words of our father, and the beginning of our journey on the HSE QUIT campaign. When we were first pitched the idea of this campaign by Dad, it was a quick and easy 'yes' from me. In my own state of numbness and denial I would have said yes to joining the circus with him if it meant it would keep his mind good and distracted from the death sentence he had received. In my opinion a lot of minds work like that in these situations – quickly jumping to do or say 'yes' to anything they believe is going to make a dying family member feel even the slightest bit better. You know, parachuting out of a plane, bungee jumping off a bridge, a very public quit smoking campaign following the last months and days of your dad's life for the benefit of the nation. The usual!

There was just something different about the way Dad thought about things and looked at life – and death, in this case. There always had been. I don't think anyone who knew him could disagree. He could always see things from a slightly different angle to the rest of us, which was a gift I most admired about him.

It wasn't long after saying yes to being part of this campaign that we were briefed on the magnitude of what we were undertaking. I realised then that Dad's proposal of this quit smoking campaign, to which I had so quickly said yes to keep him happily distracted, was not actually for his sake at all, but for all of ours. You see, Dad didn't view his cancer as a death sentence; instead, it was an opportunity.

Saying that, of course we could never have imagined the impact of the campaign – it went on to have the biggest effect on smokers in Ireland of any campaign to date. Just months after Dad passed and the adverts had aired on TV, 80,000 people had attempted to quit smoking in Ireland and visits to the QUIT website had increased from 48,000 in the previous year to 131,000. By the end of 2014, quit attempts had increased again to 175,000 and there were 45,000 fewer smokers recorded in Ireland than in 2013.

And Dad's efforts to get his message out there did not go unacknowledged by the Irish people, including our government. He received a heartfelt thank you letter from the former minister for health, James Reilly, on 1 March 2013, the day before he died. Our family also received thousands of messages from people who were touched by the campaign and had quit smoking. They could no longer thank Dad by that point, of course, though we believe he heard the messages and we remain truly grateful to the many people who got in touch with us to share their stories, sympathies and thanks, as these were a huge comfort to us then and remain so now.

Many people stated they felt like they knew him, that they could feel how genuine he was. People could relate to him, see themselves reflected in him and were devastated when he died.

The campaign has proven to be a huge success in raising awareness and helping people to quit smoking. By 2015 Dad's message had been heard loud and clear around the country.

It was even powerful enough to reach into the depths of the Seanad and be quoted by James Reilly during his closing speech on standardised cigarette packaging:

> *Many Members will know of Gerry Collins from the HSE's powerful anti-smoking advertisement. When diagnosed with terminal lung cancer, he bravely volunteered to spearhead a campaign to inform the public of the real consequences of smoking. Sadly, Gerry, a father of three, passed away from lung cancer one year ago yesterday, at the age of only fifty-seven years. I believe it is appropriate that I conclude the passage of this Bill through the Oireachtas by quoting Gerry's final line in that anti-smoking advertisement:*
>
> *'I'm going to die soon, from smoking. I'm not dying from anything other than cigarettes. Don't smoke. Don't start, and for those who have, stop.'*
>
> *The message is simple: smoking kills. We owe it to our children to protect them from this and today we do so. I commend the Bill to the House.*

Proud doesn't begin to cover it. The ads and their message were so effective that in the same year the Northern Ireland Public Health Agency requested permission to air them and has also gone on to receive extremely positive feedback from them. By December 2016 it was estimated that over 300,000 quit attempts were made in the Republic of Ireland since the ads first aired. By the time 2017 came around the HSE and GAA decided to do something that was never done before: a smoke-free day at Croke Park for the All-Ireland Hurling Semi-Final between Cork and Waterford on 13 August. It was a campaign called #HurltheHabit and was a huge success. Dad's ads were aired at half-time to a stadium of 72,000 people, something even Dad – a GAA man himself – couldn't have imagined and would have been absolutely blown away by.

The HSE QUIT campaign has had an astounding impact on the Irish people. This impact stemmed from one man's determination to promote life and insist that if you have a choice you don't choose to cut short your life, your time with your loved ones and their time with you. You choose you, you choose your family and friends, you choose life and QUIT.

I was twenty-five years old when the most important man in my life died. I know it sounds strange but I am still waiting for him to come back, to walk through the front door and say, 'Hiya, Babs!' with a cheerful smile and kiss me on my forehead. Something I took for granted for twenty-five years.

I miss talking to Dad, his bear hugs and the confidence in his voice when he would tell me that everything was going to be okay. I believed him and he believed in me. Life is different now. I cherish the rare beautiful moments in my dreams when he visits me for a stroll in places that resemble our old reality.

I tell him I miss him; he tells me everything is going to be okay and, once again, I believe him.

STEPHEN

To Dad,

It is a proud day today for me, seeing the incredible impact you have had on so many people, both in your daily interactions with people and of course through the impact of the QUIT campaign.

I wanted to share one of your favourite quotes in this book; it's a quote that continues to inspire me today:

> It is not the critic who counts; not the man who points out how the strong man stumbles, or where the doer of deeds could have done them better. The credit belongs to the man who is actually in the arena, whose face is marred by dust and sweat and blood; who strives valiantly; who errs, who comes short again and again, because there is no effort without error and shortcoming; but who does actually strive to do the deeds; who knows great enthusiasms, the great devotions; who spends himself in a worthy cause; who at the best knows in the end the triumph of high achievement, and who at the worst, if he fails, at least fails while daring greatly, so that his place shall never be with those cold and timid souls who neither know victory nor defeat.
>
> *Theodore Roosevelt*

Love you and miss you daily,
Steve

ACKNOWLEDGEMENTS

When you lose a family member to cancer you soon realise just how many people have been helping you from the sidelines. There are so many who play important roles along the way – some firmly at the forefront, some a little more in the background. Each have their own unique part to play, and whether it's a starring role or a walk-on character, they can mean just as much, but in different ways on different days.

For the friends and family I mention in my book, thank you for the roles you played and your efforts and kindness throughout the journey. For being there for Dad and for being there for us as a family, I love you all dearly.

For those who didn't get a mention in the book, I want to acknowledge you now. My dear friends, all my dad's friends and my mum's extended family: your constant support and love throughout held us up when we couldn't hold ourselves. From the bottom of my heart, thank you.

I would like to acknowledge again the HSE, the film crew, the carers, the doctors, the hospitals and the hospice. You are truly wonderful people. Thank you for caring for us.

At times writing this book felt like a very tall order, one I couldn't have fulfilled without a few people in particular:

Mum, Stephen and Ciara: I don't have enough words to express my gratitude for your support and encouragement throughout this process. I love you and I am so proud to be part of our family.

My husband, Tiernan: thank you so much for your boundless support, which never wavers. You make everything seem possible. I love you.

To my beautiful friend and fellow author Yvonne Joye: thank you for all your guidance, your emotional support, patience and help throughout. I couldn't have done it without you.

To Fidelma Browne: thank you for everything. A friendship for life forged under the most extraordinary of circumstances.

To Mercier Press: thank you for believing in my book. It has been such a pleasure working with you.

And lastly, to Dad: I feel you had a hand in this. I miss you every day and I hope you like your book.

Lisa x

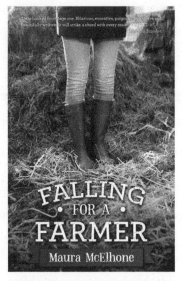

978 1 78117 604 7
Publication date: October 2018

'I was hooked from page one. Hilarious, evocative, poignant, perceptive and beautifully written, it will strike a chord with every reader. I LOVED it!' – Patricia Scanlan

After living in California for close to a decade, Maura McElhone returns home to Ireland looking to put down roots. But when she meets a handsome farmer she soon finds herself in at the deep end of a whole new way of life, from helping a sheep give birth to witnessing a slaughter, and being left in the lurch when it's time to make the silage. *Falling for a Farmer* chronicles the often humorous and sometimes sobering experiences that arise when town and country collide. This is one woman's true-life story of her journey from wide-eyed townie to full-blown farmer's girlfriend.

www.mercierpress.ie

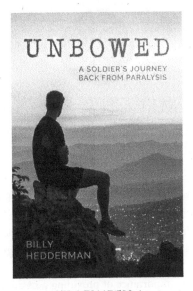

978 1 78117 593 4
Publication date: November 2018

In 2014 Billy Hedderman suffered a catastrophic injury to his spinal cord while bodyboarding on the Sunshine Coast in Australia, paralysing him almost completely from the neck down. Yet incredibly, within seven months of his injury he was running a 10km race in Brisbane in under one hour.

This is the story of Billy's injury, interspersed with the story of his time in the Irish Army, particularly his service as an officer in the elite Special Forces unit, the Army Ranger Wing, from which he took the never say die attitude that helped him prevail against all medical expectations and get back to serving as a captain in the Australian Army. A story of almost unbelievable personal resilience and mental toughness, Billy's story will amaze and inspire.

www.mercierpress.ie

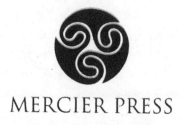

MERCIER PRESS

We hope you enjoyed this book.

Since 1944, Mercier Press has published books that have been critically important to Irish life and culture. Books that dealt with subjects that informed readers about Irish scholars, Irish writers, Irish history and Ireland's rich heritage.

We believe in the importance of providing accessible histories and cultural books for all readers and all who are interested in Irish cultural life.

Our website is the best place to find out more information about Mercier, our books, authors, news and the best deals on a wide variety of books. Mercier tracks the best prices for our books online and we seek to offer the best value to our customers.

Sign up on our website to receive updates and special offers.

www.mercierpress.ie
www.facebook.com/mercier.press
www.twitter.com/irishpublisher

Mercier Press, Unit 3b, Oak House, Bessboro Rd, Blackrock, Cork, Ireland